Morton Jim (Dept. of Anaesthetics)
2.6.83.

Current Topics in Anaesthesia

General Editors: Stanley A. Feldman
Cyril F. Scurr

5 Neonatal Anaesthesia

Titles now published

Titles in preparation

Neonatal Anaesthesia

David J. Hatch
MB, BS, FFARCS
Consultant in Anaesthesia and Respiratory Function
The Hospital for Sick Children, Great Ormond Street, London;
Sub-Dean, Institute of Child Health, University of London

and

Edward Sumner
MA, BM, BCh, FFARCS
Consultant Anaesthetist
The Hospital for Sick Children, Great Ormond Street, London

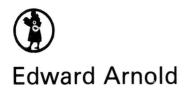

Edward Arnold

First published 1981
by Edward Arnold (Publishers) Ltd
41 Bedford Square, London WC1B 3DQ

British Library Cataloguing in Publication Data
Hatch, D J
   Neonatal anaesthesia.—(Current topics in anaesthesia).
   1. Pediatric anaesthesia
   2. Infants (Newborn)—Surgery
   I. Title II. Sumner, Edward III. Series
   617'.96798   RD139

ISBN 0–7131–4370–3
ISSN 0144–8684

Phototypeset in Linotron 202 Times by
Western Printing Services Ltd, Bristol
and Printed in Great Britain by Butler & Tanner Ltd,
Frome and London

General preface to series

The current rate of increase of scientific knowledge is such that it is recognized that '. . . ninety per cent of all the existing knowledge which can be drawn upon for the practice of medicine is less than 10 years old'.*

In an acute specialty, such as anaesthesia, failure to keep abreast of advances can seriously affect the standard of patient care. The need for continuing education is widely recognized and indeed it is mandatory in some countries.

However, due to the flood of new knowledge which grows in an exponential fashion greatly multiplying the pool of information every decade, the difficulty which presents itself is that of selecting and retrieving the information of immediate value and clinical relevance. This series has been produced in an effort to overcome this dilemma.

By producing a number of authoritative reviews the Current Topics Series has allowed the General Editors to select those in which it is felt there is a particular need for a digest of the large amount of literature, or for a clear statement of the relevance of new information.

By presenting these books in a concise form it should be possible to publish these reviews quickly. Careful selection of authors allows the presentation of mature clinical judgement on the relative importance of this new information.

The information will be clearly presented and, by emphasizing only key references and by avoiding an excess of specialist jargon, the books will, it is hoped, prove to be useful and succinct.

It has been our intention to avoid the difficulties of the large textbooks, with their inevitable prolonged gestation period, and to produce books with a wider appeal than the comprehensive, detailed, and highly specialized monographs. By this means we hope that the Current Topics in Anaesthesia Series will make a valuable contribution by meeting the demands of continuing education in anaesthesia.

Westminster Hospital London

Stanley A. Feldman
Cyril F. Scurr

*Education and Training for the Professions.
  Sir Frank Hartley, Wilkinson Lecture
  Delivered at Institute of Dental Surgery, 30.1.78
  University of London Bulletin, May 1978, No. 45, p. 3

Preface

In this volume we have tried to follow the general philosophy of the Series and concentrate on aspects of neonatal anaesthesia which are of immediate clinical relevance to the anaesthetist.

Because the differences between neonatal and adult anaesthesia largely reflect differences in physiology, we have devoted the first chapter to perinatal physiology. Wherever possible we have tried to link anatomy, physiology, pharmacology, neonatal medicine and anaesthetic practice.

For the sake of clarity, we have limited the lists of references to those we feel to be most important in each section, or those which will provide an easy guide to further study. For the same reason, we have sometimes relied more on our own clinical experience at the Hospital for Sick Children Great Ormond Street, London Group, where over 450 neonatal anaesthetics are administered annually.

Finally, we should point out that we have not attempted to journey far into the vast and expanding area of neonatal intensive care, which deserves a separate volume aimed at a wider audience. We have, however, mentioned those aspects of basic postoperative care which we believe are essential to the safe practice of neonatal anaesthesia.

D.J.H.
E.S.

Acknowledgements

This book could not have been completed without advice from many medical colleagues. We are particularly grateful to Professor Martin Barrett, Dr Ted Battersby, Dr Judith Chessells, Dr Peter Helms and Mr Jaroslav Stark of Great Ormond Street, and to Dr Ted Bennett of Chicago for correcting various sections.

We should also like to thank Lynn Baxter, Dorothy Duranti, Rita Hatch, Elisabeth Moore and Diana Newlands for help with preparation of the manuscript, Drs Christine Hall and Alan Chrispin for providing the X-rays and Ray Lunnon and the staff of the Department of Illustration at Great Ormond Street for producing many beautiful photographs. We are grateful also to the authors and publishers who have kindly allowed us to use certain Figures and Tables.

D.J.H.
E.S.

Contents

Introduction

The perinatal period, defined as the period from the onset of labour to the end of the first week of extrauterine life, is the most vulnerable period in any person's life. It is only in recent years that there has been a significant decrease in perinatal mortality (the number of stillbirths and deaths in the first week of life expressed per 1000 live and stillbirths) in developed countries. In England and Wales this number was 64 per 1000 in 1940 and fell to half this by 1960. Since then it has continued to fall slowly, reaching 23.2 in 1969 and 17.5 in 1976. This is still higher than in several other Western European countries, with Sweden having the lowest perinatal mortality at 14.3 per 1000.

Many factors contribute to reduced perinatal mortality rates, including improvements in maternal care, better conditions at delivery, efficient neonatal resuscitation, and the early diagnosis and treatment of respiratory distress. In all these areas anaesthetists have much to contribute together with paediatricians, obstetricians and paediatric surgeons. In addition, general anaesthesia in the neonatal period (the first 28 days of extrauterine life) is required for the surgical correction of many congenital malformations. Encouraging results can be obtained in this field, but early diagnosis is essential. The neonate should be transferred as soon as possible to a neonatal surgical unit, where the necessary facilities are available, including medical, surgical and anaesthetic staff with knowledge of the anatomical, physiological and pharmacological differences between the neonate and the adult.

1

Perinatal physiology

Introduction

At birth the baby experiences the greatest physiological stress he will ever have to withstand. Prior to birth the fetus lives in a protected environment and, though most organs are capable of function even weeks before full term, it is not until after delivery that the functions of the placenta are at once replaced by the lungs, kidneys and gastrointestinal tract. After birth, the baby faces a harsh environment. The delivery may have been traumatic, and effects of drugs and anaesthesia given to the mother may still be affecting the baby. After birth, organs and physiological systems develop at different rates; for example, the liver reaches maturity long before the kidneys or the central nervous system. The development of the neuro-muscular junction is related to the length of extrauterine life rather than to gestational age. During the early days of life, adaptations occur in all systems, sometimes even with a transitional stage, to fit the baby eventually for adult life. This changing pattern of function in all systems has very many implications for the anaesthetist.

Respiration

The lungs during fetal life

Before birth all gas exchange and acid–base balance is performed by the placenta, but the development of the lungs must prepare them to be able to take over full respiratory function by weeks 24–28 of gestation. The total complement of airways and blood vessels is achieved by week 16 in man but the number of alveoli present is relatively few even at term. The terminal airways, however, are fully capable of acting as gas-exchanging areas. At about week 24 of gestation, granules appear in the alveolar lining cells. These granules almost certainly represent the precursor of surfactant, the lipoprotein complex which lowers surface tension in the fluid lining of the alveoli once a fluid/air interface has developed. Without surfactant, the lungs would be unable to retain gas within them and would be unstable because the pressure within them required to prevent collapse due to surface tension is inversely proportional to their radius (Laplace formula). As areas of lung collapse, the collapsing forces increase and thus a state of unstable equilibrium exists. The quantity of surfactant which can be detected in lung

1

extracts from human fetuses increases greatly towards term and this is one of the main reasons why the older fetus has a greater chance of surviving in air than those delivered very prematurely. Surfactant deficiency is almost certainly the main factor in the development of the idiopathic respiratory distress syndrome of the newborn (RDS), though other factors such as asphyxial damage before or during birth may determine whether or not a particular premature infant develops RDS.

Recent work shows that it is possible to identify babies particularly at risk from RDS by estimation of the lecithin levels in amniotic fluid aspirated at various stages of gestation. The concentration of sphingomyelin in the amniotic fluid remains constant throughout pregnancy whilst surfactant production is accompanied by the appearance of lecithin. The easily measured lecithin/sphingomyelin ratio is used to assess fetal lung maturity. When this ratio is above 2 the risk of RDS is very small, and when it is less than 1.5 the risk is high. This information is particularly useful when premature induction of labour is being considered.

During fetal life the lungs are filled with fluid, and although the respiratory muscles contract vigorously from time to time from an early age they cannot move much fluid in and out because of the large frictional forces involved. The value of the antenatal respiratory movements is still uncertain, but in the mature human fetus breathing movements are present between 60 and 90 per cent of the time. The study of fetal breathing movements with real-time ultrasound may provide a better screening test of fetal health than biochemical estimations.

Gas transport in fetal life

The oxygen tension of fetal blood is considerably lower than that of the mother although levels of Po_2 do not vary to the same extent. Raising the maternal Po_2 by 20 kPa (150 mm Hg) only increases fetal Po_2 by 1.1 kPa (8 mm Hg), and falls in maternal Po_2 will also have relatively little effect on the fetus. Fetal blood has a greater affinity for oxygen than adult blood, which enables it to carry more oxygen in the presence of a relatively low Po_2; the oxygen/haemoglobin dissociation curve is shifted to the left (Fig. 1.1). This is due to the fact that fetal haemoglobin (HbF) is relatively insensitive to 2,3-diphosphoglycerate (2,3-DPG) which in itself lowers the oxygen affinity of the haemoglobin molecule. At a given oxygen tension, the oxygen content of the blood of premature babies is lower than at term (Fig. 1.2). A decrease in pH (Fig. 1.3) and a rise in body temperature will move the dissociation curve to the right, and conversely a rise in pH or fall in body temperature has the reverse effect. It might be thought that the increased affiinity of fetal blood for oxygen would hinder the release of oxygen at the tissues, but the simultaneous uptake of carbon dioxide shifts the dissociation curve to the right. Because the tissue oxygen tension is so low—about 2 kPa (15 mm Hg)—and because the dissociation curve is so steep, adequate oxygen delivery to the tissues is ensured.

One method of expressing the position of the dissociation curve is to measure the oxygen tension at which the blood is 50 per cent saturated. This

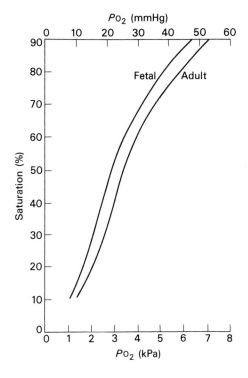

Fig. 1.1 Oxygen dissociation curves for fetal and adult blood. (From Darling *et al.*, 1941)

is known as the P_{50}. For adult blood the P_{50} is about 3.6 kPa (27 mmHg) while at birth it is around 2.7 kPa (20 mmHg). It rises slowly, reaching the adult value by 6 months of age. At birth approximately 70 per cent of the haemoglobin is HbF and total replacement of this by HbA does not occur until about 3 months after birth. The steepness and position of the fetal oxygen/haemoglobin dissociation curve are advantageous for normal fetal gas exchange; after birth, however, severe tissue hypoxia can occur if arterial oxygen tension is allowed to fall substantially. In neonatal pulmonary disease with hypoxaemia this factor is sometimes sufficiently important to justify exchange transfusion, replacing fetal blood with adult blood with its lower oxygen affinity.

Adaptation to extrauterine life

During vaginal delivery the baby's thorax is squeezed as it passes through the birth canal and up to 35 ml of fluid drains out of the mouth. As the thoracic cage re-expands at birth, this volume of fluid is replaced by the entry of an equivalent volume of air into the trachea and main air passages. Many factors stimulate the newborn infant to take its first breath, including non-specific stimuli such as sound, touch, temperature and the effect of gravity, but one of the main factors appears to be a sudden resetting of the chemoreceptors. The sudden increase in sensory activity arising at the

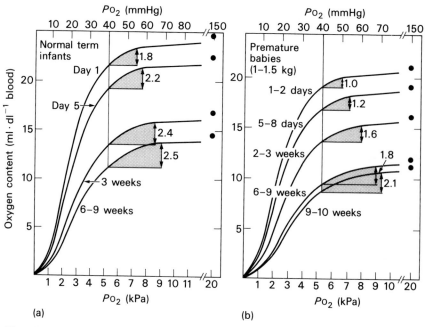

Fig. 1.2 The blood oxygen-releasing capacity at various ages from birth. (a) Term infants. (b) Preterm infants. The shaded area represents AV oxygen content in ml $O_2 \cdot dl^{-1}$ blood. (From Delivoria-Papadopoulos, Roncevic and Oski, 1971)

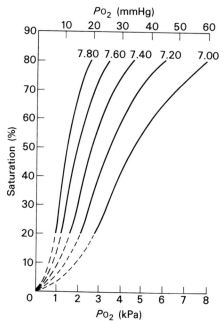

Fig. 1.3 Oxygen/haemoglobin dissociation curves for fetal blood at various pH levels. (From Hellegers and Schrueffer, 1961)

moment of birth activates the reticular system and causes a resetting of the respiratory centres, so that levels of oxygen and carbon dioxide tension which previously did not stimulate respiration now do so. The arterial oxygen tension falls during the birth process from its fetal level of about 4 kPa (30 mmHg), levels as low as 2 kPa (15 mmHg) have been reported. Increased glycogen stores protect the newborn infant to some extent from hypoxic tissue damage; CO_2 tension rises from about 6.7 kPa (50 mmHg) with a consequent fall in pH from its fetal level of 7.2. The reduction in blood flow through the umbilical vessels is also an important factor in initiating the onset of respiration, possibly by causing a sudden change in blood flow through the carotid bodies. The chemoreceptors are certainly not essential since, in experimental animals, respiration will start if they are denervated. Chemoreceptor responses become sensitive to small changes in arterial blood gas tensions early in postnatal life.

After the onset of the first breath, which may require inspiratory pressures of 70 cmH$_2$0 or more, a functional residual capacity (FRC) of 30–35 ml·kg^{-1} is rapidly established (Fig. 1.4). Remaining lung fluid is removed by the pulmonary lymphatics and lung capillaries which open up with lung expansion. A normal FRC is usually established within 60 minutes of birth. The rapid rise in arterial oxygen tension which follows the onset of respiration leads to a dramatic fall in pulmonary vascular resistance and an uptake

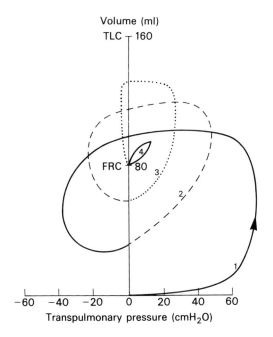

Fig. 1.4 The first four breaths. Each successive breath requires less pressure and adds increasing volume to the lungs. (Based on data from Karlberg and Koch, 1962)

of up to 100 ml blood into the pulmonary circulation. The fall in pulmonary vascular resistance with increased pulmonary blood flow, together with reduction in inferior vena caval return due to clamping of the umbilical cord, causes left atrial pressure to exceed right atrial pressure with closure of the foramen ovale. As the arterial oxygen tension rises, the smooth muscle in the ductus arteriosus constricts and closure is usually physiologically complete within 10–15 hours. These cardiac and pulmonary changes are obviously inter-related; ventilation improves both pulmonary perfusion and surfactant release, which in turn help further improve ventilation. Surfactant synthesis is dependent upon satisfactory oxygenation and acid–base state.

Respiratory function in the newborn

Over the first few hours of life the newborn infant establishes a tidal volume of approximately 6 ml·kg^{-1} and breathes at between 30 and 40 breaths per minute. Many healthy infants weighing less than 1.5 kg have respiratory rates of 50–60 per minute for the first 2 months of life. The dead space/tidal volume ratio is about 0.3, which is similar to the adult, but alveolar ventilation is approximately twice that of the adult at 150 ml·kg^{-1} per minute due to the high neonatal metabolic rate. Consequently, changes in inspired oxygen concentration will rapidly affect arterial oxygen tension. The FRC of 35–40 ml·kg^{-1} established in the first few minutes after birth changes very little throughout the newborn period. The lungs are relatively stiff at birth and their compliance (the volume change per unit pressure change) increases over the first few hours from about 1.5 ml·cmH$_2$O^{-1} to about 6 ml·cmH$_2$O^{-1} (Fig. 1.5). By the end of the first week of life, however, the specific compliance (compliance/lung volume) is similar in value to the adult. The neonatal chest wall is very compliant, so total compliance and lung compliance are approximately equal. The resistance to the flow of gases through the airways decreases from about 90 cmH$_2$O·l^{-1} per second in the first minute to about 25

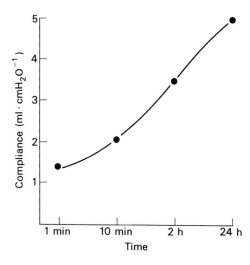

Fig. 1.5 Changes in compliance in full-term infants during the first 24 hours after birth. (From Godfrey, 1974)

$cmH_2O \cdot l^{-1}$ per second by the end of the first day, by which time an intrathoracic pressure change of only some 5 cmH_2O is needed for normal tidal breathing. The resistance of the nasal passages in the newborn is approximately 45 per cent of the total resistance. This is important in the newborn because neonates are obligatory nose breathers. The nasal resistance can be significantly increased by the presence of an indwelling nasogastric tube. Since the absolute size of the peripheral airways is small in infants, they are particularly prone to develop small airways obstruction, and airways resistance forms a larger fraction of total resistance than in the older child or adult.

The air passages in the newborn are very compliant structures, particularly in prematurity. Because of this they collapse easily during expiration, tending to trap gas behind them. That gas is trapped behind closed airways during tidal breathing in the newborn neonate is demonstrated by the relatively large alveolar-to-arterial oxygen tension difference and by the fact that FRC measurements obtained by gas dilution methods give lower results than thoracic gas volume (TGV) estimations obtained plethysmographically. This effect is most marked in the first 10 days of life (Fig. 1.6).

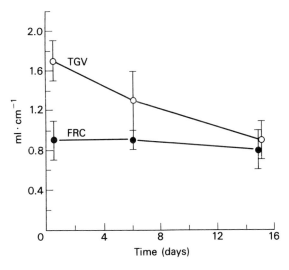

Fig. 1.6 Serial studies of FRC (black circles) and TGV (white circles) in small premature infants, showing evidence of gas trapping. (From Auld, 1967)

Relative to ventilation, perfusion is high throughout the lungs and there is a threefold increase in venous admixture. Premature babies show more evidence of maldistribution than do full-term ones.

The chest wall and diaphragm in the newborn are also very compliant structures—measurements suggest that their compliance is five times that of the lungs alone. The very compliant nature of the chest wall undoubtedly enables it to change shape dramatically during passage through the birth canal.

The diffusing capacity of the newborn infant is thought to be virtually the same as for the adult although it may be slightly lower in prematurity. The dead space/tidal volume ratio is also approximately the same as the adult value but a higher proportion of the minute volume is wasted because of the rapid rate of respiration (Table 1.1).

Table 1.1 Normal values in full-term infants compared with adults

	Infant	Adult
Weight (kg)	3.0	70
Surface area (m²)	0.19	1.8
Surface area/weight (m²·kg⁻¹)	0.06	0.03
Respiratory frequency (breaths·min⁻¹)	30–40	12–16
Tidal volume (V_T) (ml·kg⁻¹)	6–8	7
Dead space (V_D) (ml·kg⁻¹)	2–2.5	2.2
V_D/V_T	0.3	0.3
Vital capacity (VC) (ml·kg⁻¹)	35–40	50–60
Thoracic gas volume (TGV) (ml·kg⁻¹)	35–40	30
Functional residual capacity (FRC) (ml·kg⁻¹)	27–30	30
Lung compliance (C_L) (ml·cmH₂O⁻¹)	5–6	200
Specific compliance (CL/FRC) (ml·cmH₂O⁻¹·ml⁻¹)	0.04–0.06	0.04–0.07
Airways resistance (R_{aw}) (cmH₂O·l⁻¹·s⁻¹)	25–30	1.6
Work of breathing (g·cm⁻¹·l⁻¹)	2000–4000	2000–7000
Diffusion capacity (DL_{CO}) (mlCO·kPa⁻¹·min⁻¹)	6–22.5	112.5–187.5
Resting alveolar ventilation (V_A) (ml·kg⁻¹·min⁻¹)	100–150	60
Resting oxygen consumption (V_{O_2}) (ml·kg⁻¹·min⁻¹)	6.8	3.3
Arterial oxygen tension (Pa_{O_2}) (kPa)	9–10.6	10.6–12.6
(mmHg)	(65–80)	(80–95)
Arterial carbon dioxide tension (Pa_{CO_2}) (kPa)	4.7	4.7–6.0
(mmHg)	(35)	(35–45)

Gas exchange in the newborn

Oxygen consumption in the newborn at neutral environmental temperature is approximately 7 ml·kg⁻¹ per minute, which is about twice that of the adult on a weight basis. Measurements made below neutral environmental temperature will be misleadingly high because of the increase in metabolic rate in response to cold. The respiratory quotient is low in the immediate postnatal period at about 0.7, increasing to 0.8 by the end of the first week.

Studies of arterial blood gas tensions in the newborn show that the relative hypoxia of the fetus is largely corrected by 5 minutes after birth, the hypercapnia by 20 minutes and the acidosis by 24 hours. The arterial oxygen tension in the neonate remains lower than the adult value, at about 10–10.7 kPa (75–80 mmHg) and the arterial carbon dioxide tension is also a little low at about 4.7 kPa (35 mmHg). This reduced oxygen tension is thought to be due either to persistent amounts of right-to-left shunting through remaining fetal channels, to intrapulmonary shunting through poorly ventilated or unventilated areas of lung, or through small amounts of systemic blood draining into the left side of the heart from the bronchial circulation. Oxygen tension rises rapidly in the first month of life (Fig. 1.7). Although the newborn appears somewhat hypoxic by adult standards, it must be remembered that his oxygen dissociation curve is shifted to the left and therefore his arterial oxygen saturation is probably over 95 per cent, and because of the higher haemoglobin level in the newborn period the actual volume of oxygen transported in the arterial blood is proportionately higher than in the adult.

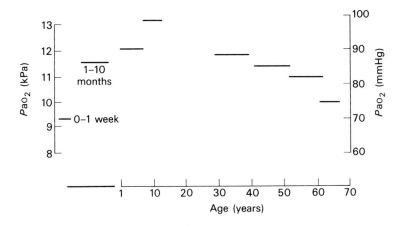

Fig. 1.7 Oxygen tensions in the newborn and at various subsequent ages. (Data from Sorbini, Grassi and Solinas, 1968, and Mansell, Bryan and Levison, 1972)

Control of breathing in the newborn

Though chemoreceptor activity is present from the moment of birth there are differences between the responses of newborn infants and adults to changes in inspired carbon dioxide and oxygen concentration.

Response to carbon dioxide. The newborn infant increases his ventilation in response to an increase in inspired carbon dioxide concentration. The slope of the carbon dioxide response curve when corrected for the smaller ventilatory capacity of the newborn is similar to that of the adult, at a value of approximately 40 per cent of resting minute ventilation per mmHg (0.133 kPa). At birth, however, the chemoreceptors are functioning at a lower arterial carbon dioxide tension and thus the carbon dioxide response curve is shifted to the left when compared with the adult, so that the increase in ventilation with increasing carbon dioxide tension begins at a lower level of carbon dioxide (Fig. 1.8).

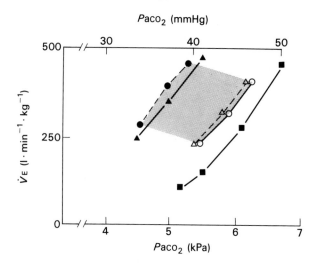

Fig. 1.8 Steady state CO_2 response curves in normal adults (black squares), normal full-term infants (black triangles), premature infants with regular breathing (black circles), premature infants with periodic breathing (white circles) and premature infants with intermediate patterns of breathing (white triangles). (From Rigatto and Brady, 1972)

Response to oxygen.   Increasing the concentration of oxygen in the inspired gas depresses respiration, and giving low concentrations of oxygen stimulates it. Unlike the effects of carbon dioxide, however, change in inspired oxygen concentration has only a transient effect on ventilation in the immediate postnatal period, passing off after about 2 minutes. This transient response develops into a fully sustained adult response by the tenth day of life. In a cool environment the newborn infant does not respond to hypoxia by increase in ventilation, and respiratory depression is seen as the only response (Fig. 1.9). After the first week of life, however, hypoxia invariably increases ventilation.

Hypoxia increases the slope of the ventilatory response to carbon dioxide and, conversely, hypercapnia potentiates the response to hypoxia.

Pulmonary reflexes.   There are two pulmonary reflexes which are important in the control of respiration in the newborn.

1. *Head's paradoxical inflation reflex.* When the lungs are inflated the infant makes an extra inspiratory effort before exhaling. This reflex, which is abolished by vagotomy, may be important in the establishment of respiration. It can be demonstrated even during deep anaesthesia.

2. *Hering–Breuer reflex.* This reflex is evoked by a more gradual inflation of the lungs than Head's reflex and consists of transient apnoea following

inflation. The premature infant attempts to inspire for longer against an obstruction than does a mature infant or adult, suggesting that inflation of the lung is necessary to inhibit inspiration. Thus this reflex may be more important in the control of respiration in the premature infant. Weakness of this reflex may lead to apnoeic spells.

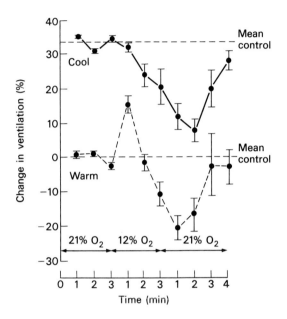

Fig. 1.9 Percentage change in ventilation while breathing air and 12 per cent oxygen in normal full-term infants in cool and in warm environments. (From Ceruti, 1966)

Periodic respiration

Pauses of up to 5 seconds occurring five or six times an hour in infants at sea level, and more frequently at high altitudes, are normal. They also occur more often in premature infants, especially during rapid eye movement sleep. These episodes of periodic breathing may develop into frank spells of apnoea, and the peak incidence of these occurs between the days 3 and 10 of life. Periodically breathing babies have a lower arterial oxygen tension than those breathing normally, though still within the normal range. They do not have an altered sensitivity to carbon dioxide, though they do not display the lowered carbon dioxide threshold described above. Periodic breathing may be abolished by increasing lung volume (e.g. constant distending pressure) or by increasing the inspired oxygen or carbon dioxide concentrations.

No constant changes in heart rate occur during periodic breathing, which appears to have no serious consequences and usually ceases by 4–6 weeks of age.

Apnoeic episodes lasting longer than 10 seconds sometimes accompanied by bradycardia or cyanosis may indicate serious illness such as idiopathic respiratory distress syndrome (RDS), septicaemia, hypoglycaemia, meningitis, cardiac failure or intracranial haemorrhage. Apnoeic attacks occur more commonly if the infant is disturbed or its environmental temperature is suddenly changed. In very low birth weight infants, both too low and too high an arterial oxygen tension may provoke apnoeic attacks, and sensitivity to these changes may vary from day to day. These infants also have a poor ventilatory response to carbon dioxide. The apnoeic attacks can be reduced in frequency by applying continuous positive airway pressure (CPAP) but in severe cases a period of controlled ventilation may be required.

The work of breathing

The work of breathing can be calculated from the area of a pressure/volume loop for an individual breath and may be subdivided into elastic work and flow resistive work as illustrated in Fig. 1.10. Work can also be calculated from formulae based on the measured compliance and resistance or from the oesophageal pressure required to produce a given tidal volume.

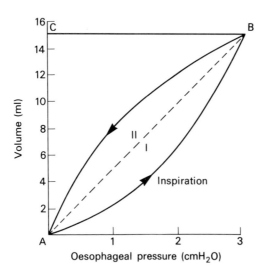

Fig. 1.10 A pressure/volume respiratory loop. Elastic work = the area of triangle ABC. Inspiratory and expiratory flow-resistive work are represented by areas I and II, respectively. Total pulmonary work work = area ABC + area I. (From data of Cook *et al.*, 1957)

Calculations of the work of breathing in the newborn suggest that its value is about 40 g.cm per breath or 1400 g.cm per minute. About 75 per cent of this work is elastic work and the rest is flow-resistive. Quiet breathing in healthy babies requires little work, and it has been calculated that a respiratory rate of 35–40 per minute is the most efficient with regard to energy consumption for the healthy neonate. Respiratory work uses about 1 per cent of the full-term neonate's energy consumption, but this may be doubled in prematurity. In respiratory disease increased pulmonary stiffness (reduced compliance) or increased airway resistance may lead to a significant increase in work, and this in turn will lead to an increase in oxygen consumption by the respiratory muscles. The work of breathing may then represent a substantial proportion of metabolic rate.

Heart and circulation

Fetal circulation

The fetal circulation has a very low pulmonary blood flow (10 per cent of the right ventricular output). The placental blood flow is high and fetal blood is oxygenated from the maternal blood. The blood with the highest oxygen content passes as quickly as possible to the coronaries and the developing brain. The ductus venosus takes umbilical oxygenated blood through the liver into the very short inferior vena cava with only minimal mixing of desaturated blood from the gut. The crista terminalis (the superior margin of the foramen ovale) directs the blood from the right to the left atrium and thence to the aorta via the left ventricle. Most of the pulmonary flow bypasses the lungs by right-to-left shunting through the patent ductus arteriosus because the pulmonary vascular resistance is higher than the systemic (Fig. 1.11).

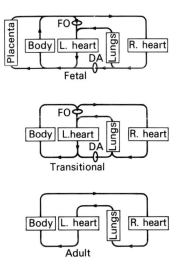

Fig. 1.11 Changes in the circulation after birth.
(From Dawes, 1968; Born et al., 1954)

DA, ductus arteriosus
FO, foramen ovale

Adaptation to extrauterine life

With the first breath and clamping of the umbilical cord, cessation of umbilical blood flow causes a reduction in right atrial pressure. At the same time, increasing pulmonary blood flow causes the left atrial pressure to rise.

This reversal of the pressure difference between right and left atria results in the closure of the foramen ovale, which eventually seals in most cases. Pulmonary vascular resistance (PVR) gradually falls under the influence of increasing arterial oxygen tension (Pao_2), decreasing carbon dioxide tension ($Paco_2$) and rising pH. This leads to a further reduction in right atrial pressure, making closure of the foramen ovale more secure. The above changes represent the transitional circulation.

Closure of the patent ductus arteriosus (PDA) by contraction of its smooth muscle begins at the pulmonary artery (PA) end under the stimulation of increasing Pao_2 after the first breath and closure of the foramen ovale. This physiological closure is completed in 10–15 hours, but permanent closure needs 2–3 weeks during which fibrosis occurs. The lack of response to Pao_2 which may cause the PDA to remain open may be due to action of prostaglandins E_1 and E_2. Bradykinin release from inactive precursors into the pulmonary circulation also contributes to the fall in PVR. The fall in temperature and pH of umbilical venous blood at birth triggers this release. After closure of the ductus arteriosus, normal 'adult' separation of pulmonary and systemic circulations is complete.

In the normal infant, PA pressure falls to adult levels in about 2 weeks, with most of the change occurring in the first 3 days.

Until the duct is firmly closed by fibrosis after 2–3 weeks, it may become patent with exposure to hypoxia, as may occur in babies with congenital heart disease or hyaline membrane disease (HMD). In infants of less than 1.5 kg who survive HMD, the incidence of PDA may be 20 per cent. This is caused not only by exposure to low Pao_2, but also by other factors such as fluid overload at a time when the oxygen mechanism for closure of the duct may not be fully developed. If the PVR is less than systemic there will be a left-to-right shunt through the duct, causing heart failure, pulmonary oedema and increased work of breathing to the extent that the duct may need urgent surgical attention. Attempts are often made to close the duct using small doses of a prostaglandin synthetase inhibitor such as a salicylate or indomethacin. Conversely, prostaglandin E, low calcium and low glucose, and a high pulmonary artery pressure all tend to maintain patency of the duct. The premature ductus is much less sensitive to the factors which cause closure so that many more remain open in these babies. Prostaglandin E may be used therapeutically by slow intravenous infusion to maintain ductal patency where this is essential (e.g. severely cyanosed infants with pulmonary atresia) until a systemic–pulmonary shunt may be created surgically.

The patent foramen ovale, though potentially patent in 30 per cent of normal adults, is held closed by the difference in pressure between the atria. The left atrial pressure rises with the increase in pulmonary blood flow following the start of respiration, and remains higher.

Cardiovascular system at birth

At birth, the heart rate is rapid—averaging between 130 and 160 per minute—and this gradually falls to around 100 by 5 years of age.

Neonates have a lower blood pressure than older children or adults.

The mean systolic blood pressure is 10.7 ± 2.1 kPa (80 ± 16 mmHg) and the mean diastolic blood pressure is 6.1 ± 2.1 kPa (46 ± 16 mmHg).

In the 2 hours after delivery the blood pressure falls slightly from an initial higher level, partly caused by compensation for the placental transfusion and partly because of the mechanisms operating during birth asphyxia which tend to induce hypertension. Maintenance of normal blood pressure is mainly due to baroreceptors in the carotid sinus and aortic arch. Afferent impulses pass through the vagus to nuclei in the brain stem. The efferent pathway passes through the sympathetic adrenergic nerves and the cardiac vagus nerve. All these reflexes function even in the premature infant.

The aortic chemoreceptors seem to be important for cardiovascular control in the newborn; hypoxia causes hypotension, vasoconstriction and variable heart rate changes, though bradycardia is the usual response.

The neonatal response to posture is less efficient and marked hypotension is seen with tilting the baby into a head-up position. If 25 per cent of the blood volume is removed at exchange transfusion there is a marked tachycardia mediated by carotid sinus baroreceptors, which does not compensate for a fall in blood pressure and which takes up to 15 minutes to recover. Peripheral vasoconstriction occurs most severely in the skin, muscles, liver, intestines and kidney. These inadequate responses suggest that the mechanisms associated with circulating catecholamines are immature at birth and the renin–angiotensin system may be more important in the neonate for the maintenance of the circulation in stressful situations such as birth asphyxia. Angiotensin II is a more powerful vasoconstrictor than adrenaline or noradrenaline. Although very high levels of angiotensin II are found after severe birth asphyxia, it may not be as important in maintaining resting blood pressure and cardiac output as it is in the stressful situation.

Stimulation of the sympathetic nerves to the heart in newborn experimental animals produces myocardial contractility comparable to that of the adult, though there is some evidence that, in the human, innervation of the fetal and neonatal myocardium may be incomplete. Thus responses elicited, though similar in sensitivity to the adult, may be of shorter duration.

Cardiac output falls during the neonatal period, with an average initial value of 400–500 ml·kg^{-1} per minute for the output of both ventricles. Initially the left ventricular output is greater because of shunts through the ductus arteriosus and foramen ovale. By the end of the first week of life, the output of the two ventricles becomes the same as fetal channels close and reaches 150–200 ml·kg^{-1} per minute. As the cardiac output falls, peripheral vasoconstriction must occur to produce the gradual rise in blood pressure seen in postnatal life.

Animal work shows that strips of fetal myocardium develop much less active tension during isometric contraction than do those from an adult. This is likely to be due to the lower proportion of sarcomeres and to the fact that these are randomly arranged rather than in parallel sequences as in the adult. However, neonatal cardiac muscle is much less susceptible to anoxia than is mature muscle if the pH is normal, thus reflecting a greater ability for anaerobic metabolism. In studies on fetal and neonatal animals, falls in cardiac output of up to 25 per cent occur in response to hypoxia (Pao_2 less than 2.7 kPa (20 mmHg)) in association with severe metabolic acidosis (pH less than 7.15).

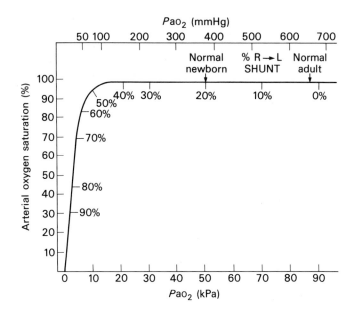

Fig. 1.12 Oxygen saturation/tension curve, showing effects of various volumes of venous admixture. Down to arterial oxygen tension of 17.3 kPa (130 mmHg), each 1 per cent of venous admixture reduces arterial tension by 2 kPa (15 mmHg). Below 17.3 kPa, the rough rule does not apply. (From Swyer, 1975)

Persistent fetal circulation (transitional circulation)

The circulation of the neonate is labile and may revert to the fetal pattern with blood flowing from the right side of the heart to the left through the ductus arteriosus from pulmonary artery to aorta and/or through the foramen ovale, if subjected to conditions which promote pulmonary vasoconstriction.

The lability of the pulmonary vasculature is a particular feature of neonatal physiology and is caused by abundant arteriolar smooth muscle, extending more peripherally than later in life. The pulmonary vasculature constricts in response to hypoxaemia, hypercapnia, acidaemia and to a low

Fio_2 via an adrenergic mechanism since it is abolished after sympathectomy.

Some infants, cyanosed after birth but without lung disease, are found at cardiac catheterization to have a high pulmonary artery pressure and a right-to-left shunt through a PDA or patent foramen ovale. This state is termed 'persistent fetal circulation' or, more correctly, 'transitional circulation' since the lungs are perfused. This state is particularly important in some babies with hyaline membrane disease and congenital diaphragmatic hernia, who may die if left untreated in a vicious circle of cyanosis, acidaemia and falling cardiac output unless steps are taken to reverse the high pulmonary vascular resistance. High inspired oxygen concentrations, sodium bicarbonate to maintain a high pH and the α-adrenergic blocking drug tolazoline have all been used, each with some success. In the newborn there is a physiological right-to-left shunt of the order of 20 per cent (adult 7 per cent). In states of persistent fetal circulation this may increase to 70–80 per cent, in which case the infant will be cyanosed even when breathing increased inspired oxygen concentrations (Fig. 1.12).

Cerebral circulation

A major cause of neonatal death is intraventricular haemorrhage. The anatomy of the circulation over the basal ganglia of the brain is unusual, with short, thin-walled and poorly supported capillaries opening at right angles into the branches of the internal cerebral vein which in turn flow into the vein of Galen at a right angle. There is a potential for venous obstruction and great surges of arterial pressure may cause rupture of the capillaries with intraventricular haemorrhage. Such surges of pressure may be caused by neonatal asphyxia or apnoea or by the osmotic effects possibly of a large bolus injection of 8.4 per cent sodium bicarbonate.

Temperature control

Heat transfer

The newborn baby loses heat in a cold environment in any of the following four ways.

Conduction

Conductive losses are generally small since it is unusual for an infant to be laid in contact with a cold surface. Conductive losses will depend on the baby's skin temperature, the area of contact and the conductive properties of the surface on which it is laid.

Convection

Convective heat loss depends on skin/air temperature gradients and air velocity. Even within an incubator the air circulation may be considerable, and small neonates may only maintain their body temperature if they are covered or if other attempts are made to reduce air currents.

Radiation

As with convection, radiant heat loss decreases as environmental temperature rises (Fig. 1.13). When the infant is in a protected enclosure, radiant loss probably becomes the most significant form of heat exchange. Radiant loss in an incubator occurs between the infant and the wall of the incubator, and between the wall of the incubator and the surrounding environment. The effective temperature in the incubator is thus affected by environmental temperature. Every 7°C difference between the inside and the outside of the incubator lowers the effective temperature in the incubator by 1°C. Radiant heat loss can be minimized by using double-walled incubators or a small Perspex shield placed over the baby inside the incubator, or by clothing the baby.

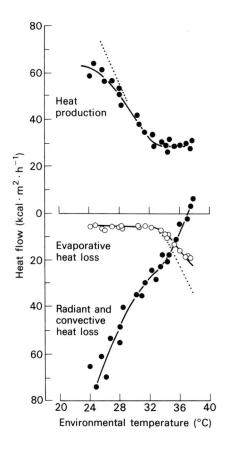

Fig. 1.13 The effect of environmental temperature on heat balance in a naked baby, weight 2.1 kg, gestation 36 weeks, when 3–7 days old, in surroundings of uniform temperature and moderate humidity. Conductive heat loss was small enough to be neglected. Heat loss by radiation and convection is large in a draught-free environment of 26°C, and falls to nothing when the environmental temperature equals body temperature (37°C). Heat production rises in a cold environment and evaporative water loss increases in a warm environment, but these changes are not enough to keep deep body temperature completely constant (the dotted lines indicate the changes that would be necessary for body temperature to remain constant). Neutral conditions are provided by an environment of 33°C. (From Hey, 1971)

Evaporation

Evaporative heat loss occurs both from the respiratory tract and from the body surface. Evaporative heat loss from the skin surface is considerable at birth when the neonate is covered with liquor amnii, as in a cold labour ward, but skin evaporative loss is not considered of great importance in normal circumstances. Evaporative loss from the lungs is increased with hyperventilation but again is not of great significance in normal circumstances.

There are several reasons why newborn babies are at particular risk from heat loss. The surface area/weight ratio is large—approximately three times that of the adult. The insulating capacity of the subcutaneous tissue is less than one-half that of the adult even for a full-term infant, and for premature infants it is even less. The ability to shiver in response to cold is poorly developed even at term and in premature infants this mechanism again is even less well developed. The main mechanism for maintenance of body temperature in the first few weeks of life is by the generation of heat in brown fat by the hydrolysis of triglycerides to free fatty acid and glycerol. This metabolic response to cold is activated by catecholamines and is blocked by beta blockers such as propranolol. Metabolism of brown fat increases metabolic rate and oxygen consumption, and any existing hypoxia is likely to be worsened. It was shown many years ago that the mortality rate of premature infants was markedly reduced by increasing the environmental temperature. The metabolic response to cold is inhibited by hypoxia, general anaesthesia, hypoglycaemia, intracranial haemorrhage and prematurity. The infant of less than 30–32 weeks' gestation appears to be unable to increase heat production to any appreciable extent in response to cold stress.

Because oxygen consumption increases in a cold environment, the ideal thermal environment will be that in which oxygen consumption is minimal. This is known as the neutral thermal environment, or neutral temperature range. This temperature range is fairly narrow for the naked newborn baby, and its mean increases from approximately 31°C at term to almost 36°C in babies with very low birth weight. The neutral temperature range is widened and lowered by covering the baby with a layer of clothing (Fig. 1.14). The metabolic response to cold continues throughout the neonatal period, though oxygen consumption is increasing rapidly, especially in the first few days of life (Fig. 1.15).

Effects of hypothermia

The main danger of hypothermia in the neonate is the increase in oxygen consumption, diverting valuable oxygen supplies from the tissues and increasing the mortality from hypoxia, particularly in RDS. Hypothermia also decreases surfactant synthesis and is associated with coagulation abnormalities. The action of many drugs, particularly the muscle relaxants and anaesthetic agents, is prolonged in hypothermic neonates.

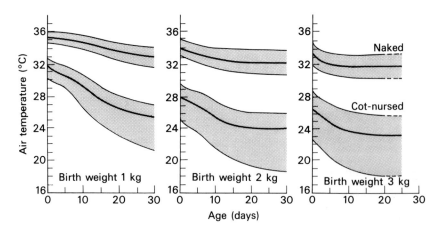

Fig. 1.14 Summary of the changes in optimum environmental temperature which occur with age in babies weighing 1, 2 or 3 kg at birth. The dark line indicates the 'optimum' temperature (at the lower limit of the neutral environmental temperature range), and the shaded area the *range* of temperature within which a baby can be expected to maintain a normal body temperature without increasing either heat production or evaporative water loss more than 25 per cent. The higher temperatures are appropriate for a baby being nursed naked in a draught-free environment of moderate humidity (50 per cent saturation), and the lower temperatures are appropriate for a baby clothed and well wrapped up in a cot in a similar environment. It must be remembered that the environmental temperature inside a single-walled incubator is *less* than the internal air temperature recorded by the thermometer; the effective environmental temperature provided by the incubator can, however, be estimated by subtracting 1°C from the air temperature for each 7°C by which the incubator air temperature exceeds room temperature. (From Hey, 1971)

Effects of hyperthermia

Although less common than reductions in temperature, raised environmental temperature can also be harmful to neonates. Increase in rectal temperature above 37°C can lead to a threefold increase in water loss by evaporation, though efficient sweating does not develop until 36–37 weeks of gestation. Neonates, including prematures, also vasodilate when their rectal temperature rises, enabling them to increase their heat losses fourfold. Oxygen consumption increases if the infant becomes restless or if his body temperature rises. Low birth weight infants exposed to raised environmental temperature or suffering from pyrexia may have an increased number of apnoeic attacks. It is known that a rise in temperature, as well as hypothermia, increases the mortality in premature infants but it is not known whether this is due to apnoeic attacks, hypernatraemia from increased fluid loss or

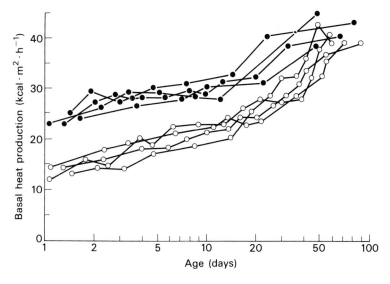

Fig. 1.15 The rise in heat production in a neutral thermal environment (standard or basal metabolism) which occurred with increasing age in four babies of 28–30 weeks' gestation (white circles) and four babies of 38–40 weeks' gestation (black circles). Heat production per unit surface area usually reaches a level comparable to that found in adults by the third month of life. (From Hey, 1971)

cardiovascular strain from increased cardiac output. These harmful effects of a raised environmental temperature, however, occur below the temperature at which oxygen consumption increases and within the neutral temperature range.

Practical considerations in the operating theatre and newborn nursery

In the operating theatre, maximum heat loss is likely to occur in the period between induction of anaesthesia and the skin incision (Fig. 1.16). It is during this period with the insertion of intravenous lines that the neonate is most likely to be allowed to become uncovered; this must be avoided at all costs, especially if the baby is premature. The operating theatre temperature should be kept as high as tolerable and it may be necessary to turn off any air conditioning. It is advisable to wrap the limbs and cover the head with aluminium foil to minimize heat loss. Anaesthesia should not be induced until the surgeon is ready, as the neonate's metabolic response to cold is suppressed once general anaesthesia has been established. Skin preparation by the surgeon should not be prolonged and should preferably be with warm fluid. Drapes should be placed over the baby as soon as possible. Infusions of blood or fluid should be warmed before administration, and for prolonged cases the inspired air should also be warmed and

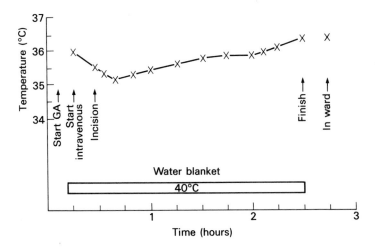

Fig. 1.16 Patient's temperature during surgery for repair of tracheo-oesophageal fistula in a baby aged 14 hours and weighing 2.1 kg.

humidified. The baby should be covered with warm Gamgee or similar material as soon as the operation is finished, and should be returned to the ward in a preheated incubator. Figure 1.14 shows the benefit of swaddling infants; this applies even in incubators because, in the UK, the maximum permitted incubator temperature is 36°C. Incubator temperatures can vary considerably around the set point and their performance can be improved by the use of servo-controlled devices. These depend, however, on the skin probe remaining properly attached to the baby, not getting wet and not being covered by anything. Overhead radiant heaters improve access to the baby and can also be servo-controlled, but they increase evaporative water loss. Servo-control mechanisms deprive the physician of the clinical information derived from changes in the infant's skin temperature.

Haematology

Haemoglobin levels

The mean cord haemoglobin in a group of premature infants is 17.5 ± 1.6 $g \cdot dl^{-1}$ and for full-term babies $17.1 \pm 1.8 g \cdot dl^{-1}$. 'Small-for-dates' babies may be rendered relatively polycythaemic by placental insufficiency. The concentration of haemoglobin may rise by $1–2 g \cdot dl^{-1}$ in the first days of life as a result of the placental transfusion and low oral fluid intake, with a decrease in extracellular fluid volume. By 1 week, the value of Hb compares with that of cord blood, but thereafter declines progressively. This phenomenon is known as 'physiological anaemia of infancy' (Fig. 1.17). Premature babies

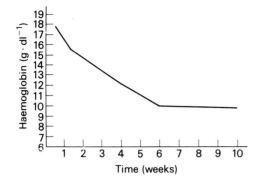

Fig. 1.17 The relation between haemoglobin concentration and age from birth in a group of infants weighting less than 1.5 kg. (From Stockman and Oski, 1978)

have an even greater fall in Hb levels—the average level being 8 g·dl⁻¹ at 4–8 weeks of life in the 1.5 kg group relative to 11.4 g·dl⁻¹ in the full-term baby. The reason for this earlier and greater fall in Hb in the premature baby is not entirely clear, though it may be related to the even shorter red cell survival time than in the term baby. The neonatal haematocrit ranges from 52 to 58 per cent (Table 1.2).

Table 1.2 Normal haematological values during the first week of life in the term infant

Value	Cord blood	Day 1	Day 3	Day 7
Hb (g·dl⁻¹)	16.8	18.4	17.8	17.0
Haematocrit (%)	53.0	58.0	55.0	54.0
Red cells (mm³ × 10⁶)	5.25	5.8	5.6	5.2
MCV (μm³)	107	108	99.0	98.0
MCH (γγ)	34	35	33	32.5
MCHC (%)	31.7	32.5	33	33
Reticulocytes (%)	3–7	3–7	1–3	0–1
Nuc. RBC (mm⁻³)	500	200	0–5	0

MCV, mean corpuscular volume;   MCH, mean corpuscular haemo-globin;   MCHC, mean corpuscular haemoglobin concentration.

(From Lubin, 1978)

The haemoglobin fall mainly results from a decrease in red cell mass (as shown using ⁵¹Cr-labelled red cells) rather than from a dilutional effect of increasing plasma volume. Red cell survival is lower in the neonate (60–70 days at term, 30–40 days in premature infants) and there is less red cell production. The reason for lower red cell survival is not known, though metabolic differences such as increased glucose consumption exist and increased glycolytic enzymes seem to confer greater susceptibility to injury. Red cell production is mediated through the effect of tissue oxygen tension on the output of the hormone erythropoietin, which is made in the liver in the fetus (kidney in the adult). The hormone is detectable in the fetal blood at birth but thereafter levels fall rapidly until between 8 and 12 weeks when erythroid activity recommences. The return to full active erythropoiesis occurs at similar minimum Hb levels even in infants born with widely differing values. The anaemia of prematurity is not seen in babies with cyanotic congenital heart disease or respiratory insufficiency. These infants continue to produce erythropoietin during the first weeks after birth and thus show no decline in marrow activity. In the healthy infant, the lower limit of normal Hb falls by about $1\,g\cdot dl^{-1}$ per week. Values of less than $8\,g\cdot dl^{-1}$ at any age require explanation, but not necessarily correction.

Factors which influence the magnitude of the physiological anaemia include the nutritional status of the infant, and supplies of vitamin E, folic acid and iron may be inadequate in the face of a rapid increase in growth later in the first year of life. The use of oral iron supplements does not prevent the early anaemia of prematurity, and indeed the anaemia is not associated with a low serum iron. Late anaemia will occur without supplemental dietary iron.

The commonest situations associated with anaemia in the neonatal period are haemorrhage (including multiple sampling for haematology or blood gases), haemolytic disease of the newborn and anaemia of prematurity.

Fetal haemoglobin

Before birth, fetal haemoglobin (HbF; α_2, γ_2 globin chains) accounts for 90–95 per cent of all Hb production and is the major haemoglobin of fetal life. The maximum rate of synthesis declines after 35 weeks' gestation and at term accounts for 50–60 per cent of haemoglobin production. The replacement of fetal by adult haemoglobin is a function of maturity of the fetus and is uninfluenced by the timing of the birth. The rate continues to decrease and at 3 months only 5 per cent of synthesis is fetal Hb. Adult haemoglobin (HbA) ($\alpha_2\,\beta_2$) synthesis increases to 35–50 per cent of new Hb at birth so that at this stage the relative concentration of HbF is 80 per cent to HbA 20 per cent. The consequence of the High HbF level and the relatively low concentration of red cell 2,3-DPG is a shift in the oxygen dissociation curve to the left (equivalent to adult blood of pH 7.6), thus favouring transport of oxygen from the maternal to the fetal circulation. Neonatal blood has an oxygen-carrying capacity at least 1.25 times that of adult blood. These two factors afford some protection for the baby under the conditions of relative hypoxia experienced during the birth process. The oxygen dissociation curve gradually shifts to the right as the concentrations of HbA and 2,3-DPG increase, so oxygen delivery to the tissues may actually increase in spite of a falling Hb.

Blood volume

The blood volume of an infant with a normal haemoglobin is estimated to be 80–85 $ml\cdot kg^{-1}$ body weight. For the premature baby a higher figure, perhaps as much as 100 $ml\cdot kg^{-1}$ may be the case. The blood volume of the newborn is more variable than that of an older infant, depending on the magnitude of the placental transfusion. Because of this wide variation, difficulties are created if blood replacement intraoperatively or otherwise is to be based on a percentage of blood volume.

It has been suggested that an alternative method of calculation based on the more constant plasma volume may be more precise. The plasma volume is generally accepted as 5 per cent of body weight (50 ml·kg^{-1}) and so total blood volume can be regarded as 50 plus haematocrit as ml·kg^{-1}.

Coagulation

Several aspects of the coagulation mechanism are defective in the neonate as compared with the adult. The infant is at risk from bleeding not only because of reduced platelet function or reduced plasma coagulation factors, but also because of the susceptibility to acute infections or metabolic disorders associated with disseminated intravascular coagulopathy.

It is widely stated that premature infants have increased vascular fragility, perhaps caused by inadequate connective tissue support of capillaries, though there is no firm evidence to support this.

Platelet counts even in the premature baby are in the same range as for normal adults, but there is evidence that all newborns have a mild transient defect in platelet function. This is without a great deal of clinical significance. Primary platelet aggregation is followed by release of serotonin and adenosine diphosphate, after which secondary aggregation occurs and this is irreversible. Neonatal platelets have lower than normal levels of serotonin and may also be mildly deficient in adenine nucleotides. The platelet defect is accentuated by phototherapy.

The levels of plasma proteins may be normal at birth, though there may be a deficiency of certain plasma proteins involved in the coagulation system. Synthesis of the vitamin K-dependent factors (II, VII, IX and X) by the liver is suboptimal until adult levels are attained after the age of 2 months. Newborns have grossly deficient stores of vitamin K at birth and deficiency will occur especially in breast-fed babies. By the second or third day of life, levels may drop as low as 5–20 per cent of the adult level before rising later in the first week of life secondary to production of vitamin K by the microflora of the colon. Minimal levels of clotting factors are seen on the second or third day of life, at which time the prothrombin time may be very prolonged. This fall after birth and the risk of spontaneous bleeding (haemorrhagic disease of the newborn) or increased surgical bleeding may be partly prevented by the administration of 1 mg vitamin K parenterally. Nowadays this is given routinely. Vitamin K does not fully correct the clotting deficiencies in the neonate, as defective synthetic capacity of the production of coagulation factors by the liver continues for the first weeks of life. Proteins produced by the liver, but which are not vitamin K dependent such as factor V and fibrinogen, are in the normal range at birth. There is no transplacental passage of clotting factors so a deficiency of any one of them is detectable from cord blood taken at birth.

The fibrinolytic enzyme system is also relatively underdeveloped in the neonate. The plasminogen level is low at term and is even lower in the preterm baby.

Jaundice

Jaundice is very commonly seen even in the normal neonate, and many factors are involved. The danger of a high level of free unconjugated bilirubin is the damage it inflicts on the cells in the basal ganglia, midbrain and brain stem, known as kernicterus and manifest by cerebral palsy, deafness and mental subnormality. The uncoupling of bilirubin from albumin is accelerated by hypoxaemia, acidaemia, hypoglycaemia, sepsis and a rapid rise of free bilirubin. Unconjugated bilirubin of $340\,\mu mol\cdot l^{-1}$ (20 mg per cent) may be the dangerous level, but lower levels can cause damage in the premature, especially if they are acidotic, hypoxic, hypoglycaemic or hypoalbuminaemic.

Neonatal red cells have a shortened life, and a high haemoglobin from placental transfusion increases the incidence of jaundice (up to 32 per cent with late cord clamping). Liver enzymes associated with bile metabolism have low activity at birth, particularly glucuronyl transferase.

Jaundice may, of course, have a pathological basis which needs investigation; increased red cell destruction is the most common cause from factors such as bacterial infection or ABO incompatibility and congenital anaemias (Fig. 1.18).

Phototherapy with a wavelength of 425–475 nm is used to decompose unconjugated bilirubin in the peripheral vessels and has reduced the number of exchange transfusions necessary, though side-effects include damage to the eyes (both retina and conjunctiva) and substantial increases in insensible water losses. Unconjugated bilirubin is decomposed by blue light, to various unidentified watersoluble products. The phototherapy also shortens intestinal transit time, thus minimizing the reabsorption of unconjugated bilirubin produced by bacterial in the gut.

Nervous system

Development of the Nervous system

At birth, the brain is relatively large, being 10 per cent of the total body weight; by 6 months of age it has doubled in size and by 1 year has trebled. Twenty-five per cent of the adult number of brain cells is present at birth. The cells of the cortex and brain stem are complete in number after 1 year of life. The cerebellum has less of its total complement at birth, but reaches its final number before other areas.

The rapid growth in the first year of life is also the result of myelination and elaboration of the dendritic processes necessary for the full complex behaviour of the older child and adult.

Nutritional deprivation during the period of the postnatal growth 'spurt' of the infant brain may give rise to impairment of cerebral development and

Serum bilirubin (mg · dl^{-1})	Birth weight	<24 h	24–28 h	49–72 h	>72 h
<5					
5–9	All	Photo-therapy if haemolysis			
10–14	<2.5 kg	Exchange if haemolysis	Phototherapy		
	>2.5 kg			Investigate if bilirubin >12 mg	
15–19	<2.5 kg	Exchange		Consider exchange	
	>2.5 kg			Phototherapy	
20 and +	All	Exchange			

☐ Observe   ▨ Investigate jaundice

Use phototherapy after any exchange

Fig. 1.18 The management of hyperbilirubinaemia in newborn infants. Guidelines are based on serum bilirubin concentration, birth weight, age and clinical status of the patient. In the presence of (1) perinatal asphyxia, (2) respiratory distress, (3) metabolic acidosis (pH 7.25 or below), (4) hypothermia (temperature below 35°C), (5) low serum protein (5 g·dl^{-1} or less), (6) birth weight below 1.5 kg, or (7) signs of clinical or CNS deterioration: treat as in next higher bilirubin category. (From Maisels, 1975)

may explain the vulnerability of the brain in inborn errors of metabolism. Certainly infants that have suffered both prenatal and postnatal undernutrition have reduced quantities of brain cells, lipids and protein and decreased dendritic connections.

There is now good evidence that newborn motor behaviour is not, as has previously been thought, entirely at subcortical levels. Cortical potentials are elicited during neonatal seizures which are manifest clinically, corresponding with the extent of dendritic growth in the motor cortex before birth. However, at birth, myelination of the nerve fibres is incomplete and reflex responses not seen later (such as the Moro reflex) may be elicited. These reflexes depend on cutaneous stimulation and the resultant action is more widespread in immature babies.

In the very young, functional and anatomical immaturity give rise to a low pain sensitivity and limited conscious behaviour. Babies generally react to painful stimuli but do not differentiate the origins of the pain.

The high incidence of convulsions in the first months of life is not fully understood, but can be attributed to a number of factors, including poor myelination, immaturity of central inhibitory mechanisms, increased water content of the brain and a higher metabolic rate. Because dendritic connections are poorly developed at birth, fits do not spread throughout the cortex as they would in an older child and thus the clinical manifestation is often fragmentary.

By 12 weeks of gestational life, motor nerve fibres reach the extremities of the limbs, but by 28 weeks, the neuromuscular junctions are more highly differentiated in the tongue and the diaphragm than in the hand. Gamma-efferent activity is less sustained than in the adult and this may contribute to the relative hypotonia of the newborn. At this stage, the muscles are functionally a uniform group, having the characteristics of adult 'slow' fibres. Early in neonatal life the 'slow' and 'fast' groups develop at the same time that fibres lose their overall sensitivity to acetylcholine and the sub-neural apparatus of the neuromuscular junction appears. Together with this, an adult pattern of sensitivity develops restricted to the motor end-plate. Indirect tetanic stimulation is poorly sustained and there is some evidence of early tetanic fade. Because of the anatomical and physiological differences which are seen, a different response to the muscle relaxants is elicited as described on p. 75.

Kidney

Fetal kidney

The kidneys produce dilute urine from as early as the third month of intrauterine life, though the excretory and regulatory requirements of the fetus are satisfactorily carried out by the placenta. The only known function of the fetal kidney is the maintenance of amniotic fluid volume: renal agenesis may lead to oligohydramnios and compression deformities. It is important to consider the possibility of absent kidneys in newborn babies with pneumothorax and pulmonary hypoplasia where amniotic fluid deficit may prevent proper maturation of the lungs. The contribution the kidneys make to fetal homeostasis must, however, be small, as infants born with absent kidneys may have normal blood urea. It is only at birth that the kidney must take up its role of excretion of the nitrogenous end-products of metabolism, and play its part in stabilizing the volume, osmotic pressure and chemical composition of the extracellular fluid.

The neonatal kidney has often been regarded as immature, but comparison with the adult kidney assumes that these neonatal and adult organs have similar tasks to perform. This is clearly not so, if only because of the effect of growth. Approximately 50 per cent of dietary nitrogen in the newborn is incorporated into new tissue, thus relieving the kidney of half of its excretory load. As will be seen below, the neonatal kidney appears to be well able to cope with the work it is normally required to perform, though it is less well equipped to counter the effects of severe dehydration, excessive water or solute load, trauma and acidosis.

At birth, the glomeruli are smaller than in the adult, but their filtration surface in relation to body weight is similar. The tubules are not fully grown and may not pass into the medulla.

Glomerular filtration rate and renal plasma flow

It is difficult to decide how to compare these aspects of renal function in neonates and adults. Whatever basis is used is largely a matter of convention and less important than an understanding that glomerular filtration rate (GFR) and renal plasma flow (RPF) increase with growth in a predictable way. For many years comparisons were made per unit of surface area, as this was thought to relate most closely to basal metabolism. On this basis, GFR is low and does not reach adult values until the second year of life (Table 1.3). RPF rises even more slowly from the neonatal value of $150 \, ml \cdot 1.73 \, m^{-2}$ per minute to adult values ($600 \, ml \cdot 1.73 \, m^{-2}$ per minute) by 24 months. It is extremely unlikely that neonatal renal function is as inefficient as these figures would suggest; since the surface area/weight ratio is three times greater in the neonate than in the adult, it may be that surface area is not the most appropriate basis on which to make the comparison. Urea is distributed fairly uniformly throughout the total body water, and it may be better to express its clearance—and functions such as GFR on which its clearance depends—per unit of total body water. Assuming an average total body water volume of 42 litres in the adult and ascribing to the infant of less than 6 months a water content of approximately 70 per cent of its weight, recalculation of urea clearance still gives infants within 1 week of birth relatively reduced clearances compared with adults.

Table 1.3 Changes in glomerular filtration rate in early infancy

| | GFR ($ml \cdot 1.73 \, m^{-2} \cdot min^{-1}$) | |
Age	Mean	Range
2–3 hours	24	3– 38
2– 8 days	38	17– 60
10–22 days	50	32– 69
37–95 days	58	30– 86
Adult	120	105–150

(From data of Edelman, 1979)

Urea clearances comparable to those of adults are, however, reached on this basis by 1–2 months of age, and considerably better ones by 2 years. This is reasonable on physiological grounds, since the protein intake of a 2-year-old child per kilogram of body water is two to three times as high as that of adults. A comparatively small amount of this protein is used for growth at this age, and were urea clearances not higher than those of adults, the concentration of urea in the body would rise.

Irrespective of the basis of comparison, the GFR, RPF and tubular reabsorption mechanisms are poorly developed in the neonate, particularly in the first week of life. Renal cortical perfusion is particularly poor, and peripheral vascular resistance is increased. In the piglet, RPF does not become normal until the end of the first month of extrauterine life, and it seems likely that it follows a similar pattern in the human. This may account for the fact that neonates suffering from birth asphyxia or severe dehydration are particularly vulnerable to renal vascular insults such as venous thrombosis. Maximum para-aminohippurate secretion and glucose reabsorption are both low in relation to GFR, there is poor reabsorption of filtered amino acids and the renal bicarbonate threshold is low. The restrained GFR probably prevents the overperfusion of the poorly developed tubules, and limits the loss of sodium and water, especially in response to water loading.

Concentration and dilution

The ability of the neonatal kidney to concentrate the urine in response to water deprivation is less than in the adult. In the first week of life the neonate cannot concentrate his urine much above 600 milliosmoles per litre ($mOsm \cdot l^{-1}$), and even when no water has been given for 3 days following birth, concentrations above $500 \, mOsm \cdot l^{-1}$ are seldom reached. This is, however, largely due to solutes such as urea being excreted at too low a rate to be concentrated, rather than to impairment of tubular reabsorption alone, and the apparent defect is less on a high protein diet. Concentrations of non-urea solutes are similar in neonates and adults.

The neonate has virtually no diuretic response to a water load for the first 48 hours after birth. By the end of the first week dilute urine can be produced, but output tails off before the full water load has been excreted.

Sodium

The neonatal kidney is poor at retaining sodium, especially during prematurity. The premature kidney leaks three times more sodium than at term, and hyponatraemia is therefore common.

Excretion of a sodium load is also poor, rising from approximately $1.5 \, mmol \cdot 1.73 \, m^{-2}$ per hour at birth to reach the normal adult value of $15–16 \, mmol \cdot 1.73 \, m^{-2}$ per hour by 1 year.

Potassium

Potassium levels are high at birth, and well tolerated. Even values as high as $10 \, mmol \cdot l^{-1}$ can occur without changes in the ECG and without treatment necessarily being required. Serum potassium levels fall gradually in the first 48 hours of life, but mainly because of a shift into the cells with correction of acidosis rather than by renal excretion.

Acid–base changes

The pH of cord blood immediately after birth is lower than that of the mother, due to intrapartum asphyxia. In the premature infant a metabolic acidosis may persist for several days (see p. 36), but in the full-term infant the pH usually rises to the normal adult level within 12 hours of birth. Metabolism of milk produces hydrogen ion in excess of bicarbonate. This is excreted in the urine as titratable acidity and ammonium ion, and is substantially greater on a diet of cow's milk than on breast milk. After the first few days of life the ability to acidify the urine is normal, but the excretion of titratable acidity is low due to low phosphate excretion, and ammonia excretion is reduced in proportion to GFR. During acidosis only a modest increase in acid excretion is possible, resulting in the rapid development of acidaemia in response to only a small increase in hydrogen ion.

Extrarenal factors affecting neonatal metabolism

Growth

By the end of the first week of life, the normal full-term neonate on a diet of breast milk may be consuming 2 g protein·kg^{-1} body weight per day. The growing infant, however, incorporates about 50 per cent of this protein into body tissues, together with water, phosphate, potassium and other substances. The phenomenon of growth thus relieves the kidney of some of its excretory load: growth has been described as 'the third kidney'. It has been shown, however, that an adequate calorie intake is essential to protect nephrectomized puppies from the development of uraemia, hyperkalaemia or hyperphosphataemia by this anabolic mechanism.

Diet

An adequate intake of carbohydrate, fat, protein, sodium, potassium, calcium, chloride and other solutes is essential for growth. Although fat and carbohydrate are completely metabolized to carbon dioxide and water, an excessive intake of other solutes (e.g. by intravenous administration) will increase the solute load for excretion, which can be approximately estimated by the equation:

Solute load (mOsm) = 4 × dietary protein (g) + dietary
Na (mmol) + dietary K (mmol) + dietary Cl
(mmol)

Table 1.4 shows that although the calorific value of equivalent volumes of cow's milk and breast milk is similar, the renal solute load of cow's milk is nearly three times as high. An infant who is unable to concentrate his urine above $300\,mOsm\cdot l^{-1}$ will be in negative water balance on an intake of $150\,ml\cdot kg^{-1}$ per day of cow's milk, and, because he is unable to complain of thirst, could become seriously dehydrated even on this apparently adequate fluid intake. Barratt (1974) has commented that for such an infant cow's milk is as sea-water for a shipwrecked sailor, causing dangerously hyperosmolar states.

Table 1.4   Representative dietary intakes and urinary excretion of infants receiving cow's milk and human breast milk, and of adults, expressed per kg body weight per day

| Per kg body weight per day | Infants | | Adults |
	Cow's milk	Human breast milk	
Water (ml)	150	150	30
Sodium (mmol)	4	1	1
Potassium (mmol)	5	2	1
Chloride (mmol)	4	2	1
Calcium (mg)	200	50	15
Phosphorus (mg)	150	23	20
Magnesium (mg)	18	6	4
Protein (g)	5	2	1
Calories	100	100	40
Renal solute load (mOsm)*	33	13	7
Urine osmolality $(mOsm\cdot l^{-1})$†	330	130	280

* Calculated from the formula of Ziegler and Fomon (1971).
† Assuming a urine volume of $100\,ml\cdot kg^{-1}$ body weight per day in the infant and $25\,ml\cdot kg^{-1}$ body weight per day in the adult.

(From Barratt, 1974)

The effect of surgery

In adults there is a well defined metabolic response to surgery and trauma, including rapid utilization of glycogen stores, protein breakdown, and the release of antidiuretic and adrenal cortical hormones, causing water and salt retention. This is also seen in the newborn, particularly after fetal distress or birth trauma, though not in the presence of renal damage. The trauma of surgery in the neonatal period does not seem to produce this metabolic response unless the surgery is major or the baby's general state poor.

Normal water and electrolyte metabolism

The total body water content of the newborn neonate is proportionately higher than the adult, due principally to a relative excess of extracellular fluid (Fig. 1.19). Normal babies may starve for up to 4 days after birth as lactation becomes established, and during the first 72 hours after birth there is usually a weight loss of 5–10 per cent of body weight. During the first few days of life, when excess extracellular fluid is being excreted, the ability of the kidneys to produce a diuretic response to further fluid intake is limited, and though this response improves rapidly it is not fully developed until 2–4 weeks of age. This limited ability to excrete a water load in the newborn period, together with low renal clearance of sodium and chloride, may lead to the retention of undesirably large quantities of any fluid administered. On the other hand, fluid deprivation in the first 72 hours of life is relatively well tolerated *in the full-term neonate with no abnormal losses*, and despite the dilute nature of the urine renal conservation of sodium and potassium is remarkably good. It will be seen below, however, that this does not apply in the premature neonate, where insensible water loss is greater, or in the presence of abnormal losses even in full-term neonates.

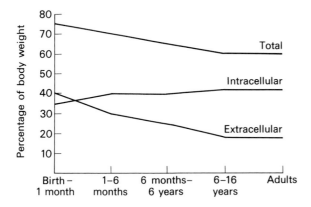

Fig. 1.19 Distribution of total, intracellular and extracellular water, expressed as a percentage of body weight related to age. (From Bush, 1971)

Water loss

Urine volume is limited mainly by the low glomerular filtration rate, especially in the first few days of life, though it is affected by variations in fluid intake and in solutes to be excreted. Most healthy infants pass urine in the first 24 hours of life and 99 per cent have micturated by 48 hours. Urine volume commences at about 25 ml per day and rises to 100–120 ml·kg⁻¹ body weight per day by the end of the first week. The osmolality falls from 400–500 mOsm·⁻¹ to about 100 mOsm·l⁻¹. Infants with water-losing renal disease are at great risk, for they may be unable to make up for their urinary water losses by drinking. Infants with abnormal kidneys may not have the usual antidiuretic and antinatriuretic response to surgery. The diuresis which follows the release of urethral valves may result in the passage of up to 1 litre of urine in 10 hours.

Insensible fluid loss in newborn neonates weighing over 2 kg is between 0.7 and 1 ml·kg⁻¹ per hour under usual environmental conditions. In premature babies, however, insensible water loss is much greater, and values between 2.5 and 3 ml·kg^{-1} per hour have been measured in neonates weighing less than 1 kg. Insensible water loss increases during exposure to radiant energy from overhead heaters, and also during phototherapy. The increase with radiant heaters varies from 50 to 200 per cent, depending on the maturity of the infant and the type of heater used; water loss during phototherapy can be minimized by careful temperature control of the infant. Insensible water loss also increases when environmental temperature is excessively high, as in the tropics, and will be affected by changes in the humidity of ambient air, though the magnitude of such changes in normal circumstances is relatively small. Water loss in the faeces is also usually small, except in the presence of diarrhoea.

Metabolism

Liver function

Before birth, most of the functions of the liver are performed by the placenta or by the maternal liver, but at birth and shortly after, the liver must take on its major role in body homoeostasis. At this time there is considerable instability as enzyme functions develop, though the liver at birth weighs 4 per cent of total body weight compared to 2 per cent in the adult. Some aspects of liver function such as detoxication and carbohydrate metabolism are poorly developed at birth, particularly in prematurity, but others such as synthesis of albumin and coagulation factors are relatively normal. Liver enzyme systems mature rapidly after birth and function at adult levels very early in the neonatal period.

Most of the amino acids essential for rapid growth of the fetus are supplied via the placenta. After birth, those amino acids which cannot be metabolized must be supplied in the diet and thus represent essential amino acids at this stage. For example, the last enzyme in the trans-sulphuration pathway for cystine synthesis is absent in the human fetal liver and thus cystine is an essential amino acid to the human neonate. It is readily available in breast milk (Table 1.5). Albumin synthesis in the liver begins at 3–4 months' gestation and increases towards term.

Table 1.5   Essential amino acids

Adult	Infant
Isoleucine	All those required by adult, plus:
Leucine	Histidine
Lysine	Proline
Methionine	
Phenylalanine	Alanine
Threonine	Cystine
Tryptophan	
Valine	

Alpha-fetoprotein (AFP) is an α_2-globulin synthesized by the fetal liver, with a maximum production at about week 13 of fetal life. If it is detectable in the serum of babies after the neonatal period, it may be a sign of hepatoma or teratoma.

A major function of the liver is to metabolize bilirubin from the breakdown of red cells and cytochromes and to excrete conjugated bilirubin in the bile. Some drugs (such as sulphonamides) displace bilirubin from albumin, which increases the concentration of unbound lipid-soluble bilirubin, thus increasing the possibility of brain damage. Glucuronide conjugation—one of the main methods for detoxification in the liver—is very low at birth. The conjugation of bilirubin is very inefficient, as is that of exogenous substances (see below). The proportion of conjugated bilirubin is slightly less in the neonate than the adult, but more significant is the fact that only 20 per cent of the bilirubin is found as the diglucuronide in the baby, the rest being the mono form. The second molecule of bilirubin is bound less freely than the first. This represents much less efficient conjugation, reflected in the low activity of the hepatic uridine diphosphoglucuronyl transferase system. Adult levels of activity are reached after about 70 days. Physiological jaundice is discussed on p. 26.

Carbohydrate metabolism

The liver plays a vital role in carbohydrate metabolism, which includes: the storage of carbohydrate as glycogen; the synthesis of glucose by the process of gluconeogenesis; the conversion of carbohydrate to fat; and the release of glucose from glycogen. There is a rapid synthesis of glycogen by the liver as fetal life comes to an end (from 36 weeks). The carbohydrate reserves of the normal newborn are relatively low (about 11 g·kg^{-1} body weight) and one-third of this is available from liver glycogen. The low birth weight baby has proportionately lower carbohydrate reserves. Energy is derived from the use of fat and protein as well as carbohydrate. The amount and availability of each 'fuel' depend on constraints imposed by immaturity of metabolic pathways, caused by lack of specific enzymes or hormones in the first few days of life. The lower the birth weight, the poorer is the carbohydrate tolerance because of deficient insulin response. In such infants, feeding within 4 hours of birth is essential.

Glucose is the main energy source during the first few hours after delivery, and the blood sugar falls rapidly. Liver and muscle glycogen stores fall. Fat metabolism then takes over.

Blood sugar levels in the normal term baby average 2.7–3.3 mmol·l^{-1} (50–60 mg per cent). For a low birth weight infant 2.2 mmol·l^{-1} (40 mg per cent) is an average random finding. Hypoglycaemia and its treatment are discussed on p. 57.

Drugs

There are four major factors involved in the handling of drugs, their bio-availability and therapeutic actions.

1. *Absorption*. Water-soluble drugs such as the antibiotics, penicillin, tetracyclines and chloramphenicol are all well absorbed after oral adminis-

tration. Ampicillin may be better absorbed in the small baby than in the adult.

2. *Distribution* is affected by many factors such as tissue mass, blood flow, lipid solubility, permeability and protein binding. The neonate has a greater proportion of the body weight as water, though this varies from baby to baby, depending on such factors as the extent of the placental transfusion. There is less fat than in the adult and the blood–brain barrier is less well developed. The markedly increased sensitivity of the neonate to the respiratory depressant effects of the opiate analgesics may be a result not only of greater quantities of the drug crossing the blood–brain barrier, but also of the increased sensitivity of specific receptors in the brain. Protein binding in the neonate is less than in the adult and there may be a greater proportion of a drug freely available for diffusion.

3. *Detoxication* takes place in the liver and relies mainly on the mechanisms of oxidation (e.g. barbiturates undergo side-chain oxidation as part of the detoxication process) and conjugation, usually with glucuronic acid. Such is the fate of morphine, salicylates, adrenal steroids, chloral hydrate, chlorpromazine and chloramphenicol. Since the enzyme activity involved in the metabolism of these drugs is poor in the early days of life, it is better to avoid their use where possible. Inefficient glucuronidation of chloramphenicol may lead to a build-up of its blood levels, resulting in the 'grey' syndrome of cardiovascular collapse and typical grey appearance.

4. *Excretion.* The neonatal GFR is only 30–40 per cent of the adult value, though adult levels are attained in the first year of life. Thus drugs excreted unchanged by the kidneys will have a prolonged action because of the delayed excretion. Drugs such as digoxin and gentamicin treated in this way must have serum levels monitored carefully after several days of administration.

Acid–base state

Blood gases taken from the cord blood show a combined respiratory and metabolic acidosis; for example, pH 7.26, $Paco_2$ 7.3 kPa (55 mmHg). Pao_2 2.7 kPa (20 mmHg).

After clamping of the cord, the $Paco_2$ falls to below normal and stays between 4.3 and 4.8 kPa (32–36 mmHg) for a few days before rising towards 5.3 kPa (40 mmHg) by 2–3 weeks of age (Fig. 1.20).

The pH rapidly rises from values found in cord blood to about 7.30 and stays for 2–3 weeks between 7.34 and 7.36 before values of over 7.38 are found. A mild metabolic acidosis may persist for weeks, especially in a premature baby fed on cow's milk. Full correction must wait for renal maturation. Changes in pH can be expected to influence potassium and calcium metabolism and the $Paco_2$. It is usual to give half the calculated dose initially and then re-assess the situation. Correction of base deficit greater than 5 should be undertaken using the formula:

$$\text{ml } 8.4 \text{ per cent sodium bicarbonate} = \frac{\text{kg wt}}{3} \times \text{base deficit}$$

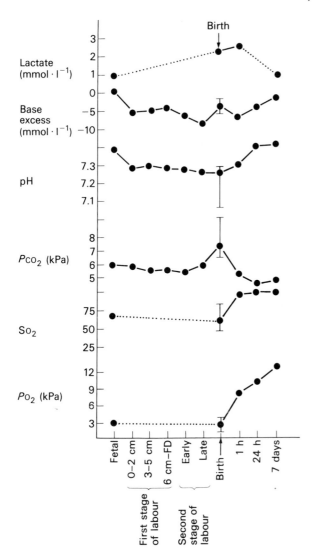

Fig. 1.20 Changes occurring in fetal and newborn blood over the perinatal period (—). FD, full dilatation of cervix (—). (From Swyer, 1971)

The sodium bicarbonate solution has an osmolality of 2000 mOsm·l^{-1} and if given quickly may cause cellular damage, especially of the brain, and has been incriminated in the production of intraventricular cerebral haemorrhage.

Metabolic acidosis in the newborn commonly results from asphyxia or circulatory failure from a variety of causes. In asphyxial acidosis of the newborn, circulatory failure may occur because of interference with the breakdown of glycogen in the heart under anaerobic conditions. The effects on the brain can be equally disastrous and may be irreversible.

Monitoring of acid–base state must be frequent if adequate treatment is to be undertaken. Fresh arterial blood is preferable since it also gives information about alveolar ventilation and alveolar–arterial oxygen difference ($A-aDo_2$) may be calculated.

Calcium

The fetus acquires most of its calcium stores in the last 12 weeks of gestation, and at birth the calcium and phosphate levels are higher than maternal. There is active transport of calcium ions from the mother to the fetus and the phosphate is high because of the relative hypoparathyroidism of the fetus. As expected, low birth weight babies have deficient stores of calcium.

After birth, plasma phosphate levels rise because of a low GFR and parathyroid hormone deficiency which takes over 48 hours to rise to detectable levels. The high plasma phosphate depresses the serum Ca^{2+} level. An additional factor causing hypocalcaemia at birth is the poor conversion of vitamin D to its active metabolite. High levels of glucocorticoids also depress serum calcium.

Hypocalcaemia is discussed on p. 58.

References and further reading

General

Davis, J. A. and Dobbing, J. (1974). *Scientific Foundations of Paediatrics.* Heinemann Medical, London.

Davies, P. A., Robinson, R. J., Scopes, J. W., Tizard, J. P. M. and Wigglesworth, J. S. (1972). *Medical Care of Newborn Babies.* Clinics in Developmental Medicine, no. 44/45. Heinemann Medical, London.

Dawes, G. S. (1968). *Foetal and Neonatal Physiology.* Year Book Medical, Chicago.

Dubowitz, L. M., Dubowitz, V. and Goldberg, C. (1970). Clinical assessment of gestational age in the newborn infant. *Journal of Pediatrics* **77,** 1.

Mirkin, B. L. (1975). Perinatal pharmacology: placental transfer, fetal localization and neonatal disposition of drugs. *Anesthesiology* **43,** 156.

Rawlings, G., Reynolds, E. O. R., Stewart, A. and Strang, L. B. (1971). The changing prognosis of very low birth weight. *Lancet* **i,** 516.

Roberton, N. R. C. (1979). Perinatal physiology. In: *Clinical Paediatric Physiology.* Ed. by S. Godfrey, and J. D. Baum. Blackwell Scientific, Oxford.

Swyer, P. R. (1975). *The Intensive Care of the Newly Born. Physiological principles and practice.* Monographs in Paediatrics, vol. 6. S. Karger, Basel; Wiley, Chichester.

Symposium on the Neonatal Period. (1977). *British Journal of Anaesthesia* **49,** 1.

Respiration

Auld, P. A. M. (1976). Pulmonary transition from fetal life. In: *Reviews in Perinatal Medicine*. Ed. by E. M. Scarpelli and E. V. Cosmi. University Park Press, Baltimore.

Ceruti, E. (1966). Chemoreceptor reflexes in the newborn. *Pediatrics* **37**, 556.

Cook, C. D., Sutherland, J. M., Segal, S., Cherry, R. B., Mead, J., McIlroy, M. B. and Smith, C. A. (1957). Studies of respiratory physiology in the newborn infant. III. Measurements of mechanics of respiration. *Journal of Clinical Investigation* **36**, 440.

Darling, R. C., Smith, C. A., Asmussen, E. and Cohen, F. M. (1941). Some properties of human fetal and maternal blood. *Journal of Clinical Investigation* **20**, 739.

Dawes, G. S., Fox, H. E., Leduc, B. M., Liggins, G. C. and Richards, R. T. (1972). Respiratory movements and rapid eye movements during sleep in the foetal lamb. *Journal of Physiology* **220**, 119.

Delivoria-Papadopolous, M., Roncevic, N. P. and Oski, F. A. (1971). Postnatal changes in oxygen transport of term, premature and sick infants. *Pediatric Research* **5**, 235.

Godfrey, S. (1974). Growth and development of the respiratory system—functional development. In: *Scientific Foundations of Paediatrics*. Ed. by J. A. Davis and J. Dobbing. Heinemann Medical, London.

Hellegers, A. E. and Schrueffer, J. J. P. (1961). Nomograms and empirical equations relating to oxygen tension, percentage saturation and pH in maternal and fetal blood. *American Journal of Obstetrics and Gynecology* **81**, 377.

Karlberg, P. and Koch, G. (1962). Respiratory studies in newborn infants. III. Development of mechanics of breathing during the first week of life. A longitudinal study. *Acta Paediatrica Scandinavica* Suppl. 135. p. 121.

Mansell, A., Bryan, A. C. and Levison, H. (1972). Airway closure in children. *Journal of Applied Physiology* **33**, 711.

Nelson, N. M. (1966). Neonatal pulmonary function. *Pediatric Clinics of North America* **13**, 769.

Rigatto, H. and Brady, J. P. (1972). Periodic breathing and apnea in preterm infants. *Pediatrics* **50**, 202.

Sorbini, C. A., Grassi, V. and Solinas, E. (1968). Arterial oxygen tension in relation to age in healthy subjects. *Respiration* **25**, 3.

Stocks, J. and Godfrey, S. (1977). Specific airway conductance in relation to post conceptional age during infancy. *Journal of Applied Physiology* **43**, 144.

Strang, L. B. (1978). *Neonatal Respiration*. Blackwell Scientific, Oxford.

Heart and circulation

Born, G. V. R., Dawes, G. S., Mott, J. C. and Widdicombe, J. G. (1954). Changes in the heart and lungs at birth. *Cold Harbour Symposia on Quantitative Biology*, **19**, 102.

Downing, S. E. (1970). Metabolic and reflex influences on cardiac function in the newborn. In: *Pathophysiology of Congenital heart Disease.* Ed. by F. H. Adams, H. J. C. Swan and E. V. Hall. University of California Press, Los Angeles.

Macartney, F. J. (1979). Heart and circulation. In: *Clinical Paediatric Physiology.* Ed. by S. Godfrey and J. D. Baum. Blackwell Scientific Oxford.

Rudolph, A. M. and Heymann, M. A. (1974). Fetal and neonatal circulation and respiration. *Annual Review of Physiology* **36**, 187.

Temperature control

Bennett, E. J., Patel, K. P. and Grundy, E. M. (1977). Neonatal temperature and surgery. *Anesthesiology* **46**, 303.

Cross, K. W., Flynn, D. M. and Hill, J. R. (1966). Oxygen consumption in normal newborn infants during moderate hypoxia in warm and cool environments. *Pediatrics* **37**, 565.

Dawkins, M. J. R. and Hull, D. (1964). Brown adipose tissue and the response of newborn rabbits to cold. *Journal of Physiology* **172**, 216.

Goudsouzian, N. G., Morris, R. H. and Ryan, J. F. (1973). The effects of a warming blanket on the maintenance of body temperature in anesthetized infants and children. *Anesthesiology* **39**, 351.

Hey, E. N. (1971). The care of babies in incubators. In: *Recent Advances in Paediatrics,* 4. Ed. by D. Gairdner and D. Hull. Churchill Livingstone, Edinburgh and London.

Lewis, R. B., Shaw, A. and Etchells, A. H. (1973). Contact mattress to prevent heat loss in neonatal and paediatric surgery. *British Journal of Anaesthesia* **45**, 919.

Meyers, M. B. and Oh, T. H. (1976). Prevention of hypothermia during cystoscopy in neonates. *Anesthesia and Analgesia* **55**, 592.

Silverman, W. A., Fertig, J. W. and Berger, A. P. (1958). The influence of the thermal environment upon the survival of newly born premature infants. *Pediatrics* **22**, 876.

Haematology

Bellingham, A. J. and Grimes, A. J. (1973). Red cell 2,3-diphosphoglycerate. *British Journal of Haematology* **25**, 555.

Burman, D. and Morris, A. F. (1974). Cord haemoglobin in low birth weight infants. *Archives of Disease in Childhood* **49**, 382.

Chessells, J. M. (1979). Blood formation in infancy. *Archives of Disease in Childhood* **54**, 831.

Glader, B. E. (Ed.) (1978). *Perinatal Haematology.* Clinics in Haematology, no. 7. Saunders, Eastbourne and Philadelphia.

Lubin, B. (1978). Neonatal anaemia secondary to blood loss. In: *Perinatal Haematology.* Ed. by B.E. Glader. Clinics in Haematology, no. 7. Saunders, Eastbourne and Philadelphia.

Maisels, M. (1975). The management of hyperbilirubinaemia in newborn infants. In: *Neonatology: pathophysiology and management of the newborn.* Ed. By G. B. Avery. Lippincott, Philadelphia and London.

Stockman, J. A. and Oski, F. A. (1978). Physiological anaemia of infancy and the anaemia of prematurity. In: Perinatal Haematology. Ed. by B. E. Glader. Clinics in Haematology, no. 7. Saunders, Eastbourne and Philadelphia.

Nervous system

Green, S. H. (1979). Neurophysiology. In: *Clinical Paediatric Physiology.* Ed. by S. Godfrey and J. D. Baum. Blackwell Scientific, Oxford.

Kidney

Barratt, T. M. (1974). The nephrological background to urology. In *Encyclopaedia of Urology*, vol. 15, Suppl. Ed. by D. I. Williams, Springer Verlag, Heidelberg.

Bush, G. H. (1971). Intravenous therapy in paediatrics. *Annals of the Royal College of Surgeons of England* 49, 92.

Edelman, C. M. Jr (1979). Physiologic adaptations required of a newborn's kidney. *Contributions to Nephrology* **15**, 1.

Hey, E. N. and Katz, G. (1969). Evaporative water loss in the newborn baby. *Journal of Physiology* **200**, 605.

Jones, R. W. A., Rochefort, M. J. and Baum, J. D. (1976). Increased insensible water loss in newborn infants nursed under radiant heaters. *British Medical Journal* **2**, 1347.

McCance, R. A. and Young W. F. (1941). Secretion of urine by newborn infants. *Journal of Physiology* **99**, 265.

Roy, R. N. and Sinclair, J. C. (1975). Hydration of the low birth weight infant. *Clinical Perinatology* **2**, 393.

Smith, C. A. and Nelson, N. M. (Eds) (1976). *The Physiology of the Newborn Infant*, 4th edn. Charles C. Thomas, Springfield, Illinois.

Ziegler, E. E. and Foman, S. J. (1971). Fluid intake, solute load and water balance in infancy. *Journal of Pediatric Surgery* **78**, 561.

Metabolism

Dawes, G. S. (1968). Fetal blood gas homeostasis during development. Symposium on life before birth. *Proceedings of the Royal Society of Medicine* **61**, 1227.

Oliver, T. K., Demis, J. A. and Bates, G. D. (1961). Serial blood gas tensions and acid–base balance during the first hour of life in human infants. *Acta Paediatrica Scandinavica* **50**, 346.

Swyer, P. R. (1971). Special physiological and physiopathological considerations. In: *Care of the Critically Ill Child.* Ed. by R. S. Jones and J. B. Owen-Thomas. Edward Arnold, London.

2

The surgical neonate

Transportation

The regional care of critically ill newborn babies in modern intensive care units with physicians, surgeons and anaesthetists trained to deal with their problems has created a need for sophisticated transport systems. Transport incubators (Fig. 2.1) are now in common use and babies are daily transferred long distances, even in aircraft and helicopters.

Incubators must provide good visibility, immediate access and a constant neutral thermal environment. It must be possible to control the administration of oxygen, usually with a head hood.

If the thermal environment cannot be well maintained, the baby should be swaddled in a polyurethane-lined aluminium foil wrap which will give some protection against heat loss. Most transporting incubators provide a means

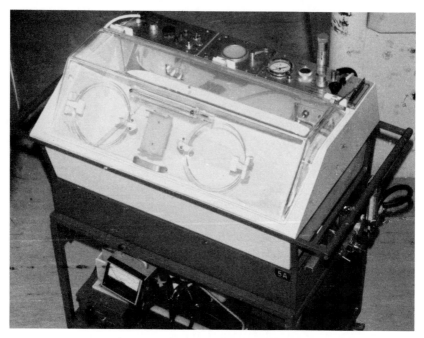

Fig. 2.1 A transport incubator (Vickers Medical).

of mechanical ventilation for those babies in respiratory failure. The supply of compressed gas and battery power must be adequate for the journey.

Before transfer, an intravenous cannula should be in place, providing secure access for intravenous administrations. A nasogastric tube must be passed in all babies with suspected intestinal obstruction, and the stomach contents aspirated at frequent intervals throughout the journey. The trachea of an infant with severe respiratory distress must be intubated before departure so that assisted ventilation may take place during the journey. The endotracheal tube must be secured very firmly indeed, as it is extremely difficult to prevent dislodgement or kinking during transport. A clear airway is essential at all times, so suction catheters and suction apparatus must be at hand. A self-inflating manual bag system such as the Ambu is necessary, as is intubation equipment. It is usual to take a prepacked kit of equipment and drugs for resuscitation on all such journeys.

Ideally, monitoring of the baby should include ECG, as listening to the heart sounds using a stethoscope may be difficult because of the noise and motion of transport. Battery-powered instruments are now available for this purpose. Continuous monitoring of the baby's temperature is also useful.

The incubator must have a means of securing the baby inside it, and must itself be secured in case of sudden movements of the ambulance or aircraft.

With the help of this equipment and careful monitoring, it should be possible to transfer even the most sick infants long distances with the minimum of disturbance. It is usual for the baby to be accompanied by a qualified nurse and a member of the medical staff skilled in intubation and resuscitation techniques.

One published series (Blake *et al.*, 1975) describes 222 patients transported over a 50-mile radius: 40 per cent of the patients were clinically improved during the journey; 56 per cent were stable and only 4 per cent deteriorated.

Preoperative assessment and management

Introduction

All neonates must be carefully assessed by the anaesthetist preoperatively. It may be necessary to explain to parents what anaesthesia in this age group involves. All babies are accurately weighed on admission and a full history and clinical examination undertaken.

Many congenital defects are multiple and a baby presenting for surgery for one defect could well have others with implications for the anaesthetist. Fourteen per cent of babies with cleft lip and 33 per cent of those with a cleft palate have other congenital abnormalities such as the Pierre Robin syndrome of micrognathia and glossoptosis; babies with Down's and Edwards' syndromes may have congenital heart disease.

The anaesthetist will be alerted to obvious intubation difficulties as seen with Pierre Robin, Treacher-Collins or the Klippel–Feil syndromes.

Feeds may be given to the baby until 4 hours preoperatively, though the last feed is better given as clear dextrose rather than milk. A nasogastric tube should be passed in any sick baby, especially those with intestinal obstruction. Gastric distension is a very common problem in infancy with acidosis and hypoxaemia as predisposing causes. There is a risk of regurgitation. Pulmonary aspiration, elevation of the diaphragm and basal atelectasis may also prejudice normal respiratory function. Oesophageal motility is reduced in the newborn, especially in the lower third, so some degree of reflux occurs continuously. The cardio-oesophageal sphincter mechanism does not develop until the end of the first year. Gastric motility may be low and up to 40 per cent of any feed may still be in the stomach 2 hours later, depending on the type of fluid (breast milk passes into the intestine more rapidly), the position of the baby (more rapid emptying if the baby is prone) and the fitness of the baby. Gastric emptying times are markedly increased in premature and sick babies. The nasogastric tube should be left to drain freely and the equivalent volume of normal saline should be given intravenously to replace the loss. The tube must be aspirated before anaesthesia and left unclamped. Too large a nasogastric tube might cause respiratory obstruction in infants, as they are obligatory nose breathers.

If possible, the baby should be taken to theatre in optimum condition in an incubator when the body temperature is normal, adequate hydration and blood volume ensured, and when all the necessary investigations and x-rays have been performed.

Prematurity

An assessment of the degree of prematurity must be made because of the profound anaesthetic and postoperative implications involved. Infants born before 37–38 weeks and with weights of less than 2.5 kg exhibit physiological immaturity compared with the term baby. Most of the problems have been discussed more fully elsewhere. Reduced hepatic function is shown by jaundice and by lower and unstable blood sugar levels. There are fewer functioning nephrons and renal clearances are diminished. Periodic respiration, including apnoea, affects 40 per cent of premature infants although this responds to the constant distending pressure of CPAP.

Greater susceptibility to infections is caused by less efficient neutrophils and lower antibody titres than in term babies. Premature babies are particularly sensitive to sedatives and anaesthetic agents, including the non-depolarizing muscle relaxants, and the mechanisms whereby the trachea is protected from soiling by aspirated material are reduced. Low birth weight babies are susceptible to retrolental fibroplasia caused by retinal vasospasm, which in turn is caused by excessive oxygen tension in arterial blood reaching the retina. An arterial oxygen tension (Pao_2) of 10.7 ± 0.7 kPa (80 ± 5 mmHg) is considered safe. Careful monitoring of inspired oxygen and arterial Pao_2 is mandatory in the low birth weight baby. During anaesthesia, care must be taken with inspired oxygen concentrations in this age group and nitrous oxide/oxygen or air/oxygen mixtures used. The premature baby is unable to maintain its own body temperature unless nursed in a neutral thermal environment. Care must be taken not to overload the circulation with fluids. All volumes given, especially those involving intravenous anaesthetic drugs diluted for use, must be accounted for on fluid balance records.

Respiration

The signs of respiratory failure include dyspnoea and tachypnoea, oxygen dependency and apnoeic attacks. Changes in blood gases may be found and pathological changes in the chest X-ray occur. A discussion of the detailed assessment of respiratory failure may be found on p. 150. Preoperative respiratory failure is usually a sign that respiratory support will be necessary postoperatively, and often this is most satisfactorily started before the operation. Oxygen therapy is discussed on p. 156, and respiratory support on p. 160.

Hyaline membrane disease

Perhaps the commonest medical condition involving pulmonary pathology in the neonate is hyaline membrane disease (surfactant deficiency, idiopathic respiratory distress syndrome). This is often seen as a complication of prematurity in the surgical neonate.

The condition occurs in 1 per cent of all live births and 1 in 3 of all premature births, and is caused by a relative deficiency of lung surfactant associated with prematurity. The severity is increased by interference with surfactant synthesis in type II alveolar cells by immaturity or by hypoxia or asphyxia in the neonatal period.

The main clinical features are tachypnoea, dyspnoea (with grunting respiration as the infant attempts to produce its own constant distending pressure), poor air entry, cyanosis and tachycardia. The chest X-ray shows a typical uniform opacity in the lung fields with an air bronchogram (Fig. 2.2).

Surfactant deficiency prevents the formation of a functional residual capacity of air by failing to stabilize small air spaces at the end of expiration. A disordered ventilation/perfusion ratio causes hypoxaemia and pulmonary vascular resistance is raised by vasoconstriction, itself made worse by hypoxia, acidosis and hypercapnia. Tachypnoea, combined with stiffness of the lungs, increases the work of breathing by up to ten times. Right-to-left shunts through the ductus arteriosus or patent foramen ovale increase the arterial hypoxaemia. Reduced oxygenation to the heart impairs its function and consequently other organs suffer reduced perfusion. Metabolic acidosis will follow and a vicious circle is set up (Fig. 2.3). Careful respiratory support involving the use of constant distending pressure or intermittent positive pressure ventilation (IPPV) with reversed inspiratory/expiratory time ratios (up to 2 : 1), and positive end-expiratory pressure (PEEP) may be required. Limiting inflation pressures to 30 cmH$_2$O preferably with a pressure generator, reduces the risk of bronchopulmonary dysplasia. Those patients who come to surgery will usually need IPPV and great attention to metabolic and respiratory functions postoperatively.

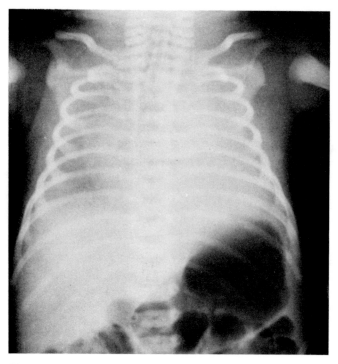

Fig. 2.2 Acute hyaline membrane disease. X-ray showing bilateral air bronchograms.

Meconium aspiration and perinatal pneumonia

Other pulmonary problems include meconium aspiration and perinatal pneumonia. The latter is the cause of 5–10 per cent of perinatal deaths; the infection is usually derived from the mother, with prolonged rupture of the membranes. Patients with cystic fibrosis (meconium ileus), congenital heart disease and prematurity are particularly susceptible. Aspiration pneumonitis, frequently complicated by infection, may be associated with inco-ordination of the swallowing mechanism, as is seen in prematurity, brain damage and with depression of consciousness or with conditions such as tracheo-oesophageal fistula, cleft palate or hiatus hernia. The infection must be dealt with properly and effectively before further lung damage ensues. The organisms involved are often Gram-negative ones such as *E. coli* or *Klebsiella*.

It is often advisable to start antibiotic therapy on clinical suspicion of infection, though bacteriological confirmation must be sought and the antibiotic sensitivities determined. Blood, urine and cerebrospinal fluid are sent for bacteriological examination as part of the initial screening tests.

Suitable antibiotics for the neonate to combat the common organisms found in this condition include cloxacillin 25 mg·kg⁻¹ 8-hourly gentamicin 2 mg·kg⁻¹ 8-hourly and ampicillin 50 mg·kg⁻¹ 8-hourly.

Congenital infections are rare, but important. Rubella has a teratogenic effect, cytomegalovirus causes encephalitis with seizures and liver damage, and herpes and respiratory syncytial viruses cause severe pneumonia.

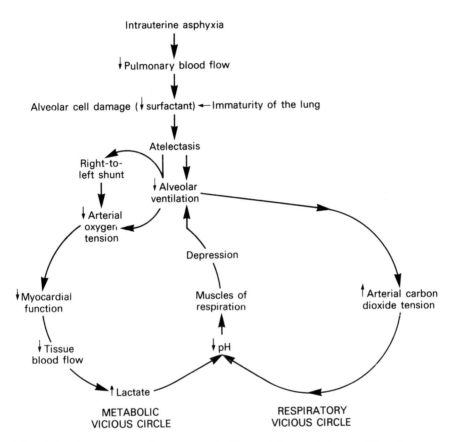

Fig. 2.3 Diagrammatic representation of the aetiology of hyaline membrane disease and its pathophysiological consequences. (From Swyer, 1975)

Active acute respiratory infections of any kind are an indication for delay of any but the most urgent operation. Lower respiratory infection is a very common sequel to upper respiratory tract infection after anaesthesia, as is a high incidence of laryngeal spasm during induction or emergence from anaesthesia.

Heart and circulation

Signs of failure

The management of newborn infants with congenital heart disease is mainly concerned with the treatment of hypoxia and congestive cardiac failure (Fig. 2.4).

Congestive cardiac failure is associated with tachypnoea and tachycardia with a gallop rhythm. Signs of raised venous pressure include a full fontanelle, cardiac enlargement and hepatomegaly palpable below the costal margin. Oedema is not a sign of cardiac failure in the newborn, though unusual weight gain may be found. Cardiac failure is also seen with cardiac malformations of the cyanotic type, when cyanosis will be unrelieved by an increased inspired oxygen concentration.

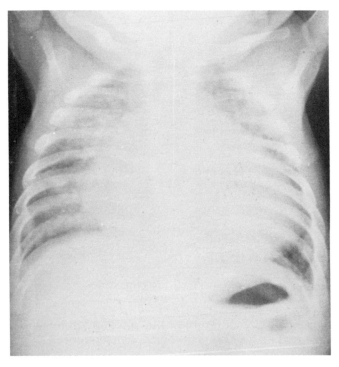

Fig. 2.4   Cardiac failure. X-ray showing large heart and congested lung fields.

Causes of failure

Lesions presenting predominantly with cardiac failure include coarctation of the aorta, ventricular septal defect, aortic stenosis and patent ductus arteriosus (PDA), and those presenting with cyanosis and failure include transposition of the great vessels, total anomalous pulmonary venous drainage and truncus arteriosus. (See Chapter 4 for discussion of cardiac surgery.)

Treatment of failure

Cardiac failure should be treated preoperatively, if necessary using digoxin 0.05 mg·kg^{-1} as a total digitalizing dose divided into three doses per 24 hours by intramuscular or intravenous injection. Maintenance is with digoxin, one-fifth of the total dose divided into two daily doses. Frusemide 1 mg·kg^{-1} intravenously as necessary may be given if the cardiac failure is severe. Because digoxin toxicity is intensified by hypokalaemia, digoxin levels and serum potassium should be measured during maintenance therapy. Potassium supplements may be necessary.

The ECG should be checked before the third dose of digoxin is given. Other treatments include correction of acidosis, oxygen therapy and possibly inotropic support by infusions of dopamine or isoprenaline as described on p. 132. Patients with cardiac lesions need antibiotic cover for surgery (see p. 195 for dosage).

Sclerema

Sclerema is a condition in which changes occur in the subcutaneous tissues of the neonate, making them feel hard and waxy. The first signs usually appear over the limbs and then extend to the trunk and the face. It may be present at birth if the mother is toxaemic, but is more usually seen by the fourth day in cases of severe asphyxia, hypothermia, sepsis, hyaline membrane disease or congenital heart disease. The condition is related to peripheral circulatory failure, ischaemia and hypothermia. Its presence worsens the prognosis of the primary condition, especially if the sclerema is extensive, when the mortality may be as great as 75 per cent. Scleremic infants are very sick, lethargic, unable to suck and may develop respiratory failure. Pathological changes of inflammation, oedema and thickening of connective tissue bands are found. Corticosteroids are usually given (prednisone 1 mg·kg^{-1} 8-hourly) though it is uncertain if they affect the final outcome of the condition. Peripheral circulatory failure must be treated by intravenous infusions of crystalloid, blood or plasma. Exchange transfusion may be necessary to help the haemoglobin to give up oxygen in the periphery. Gentamicin is the antibiotic of choice for use in this condition.

Haematology

Haemoglobin levels

The preoperative haemoglobin level should be at least 10 g·dl^{-1}, though higher levels are usually to be expected. There is no problem with sickle cell disease in the neonatal age group.

The aim of correcting anaemia should be to raise the level to $12\ \mathrm{g\cdot dl^{-1}}$ using a formula such as the following.

Subtract the patient's haemoglobin from the desired level (usually 12) to find the required amount of $\mathrm{Hb\cdot dl^{-1}}$ of blood volume. This figure is multiplied by the blood volume to find the actual grams of haemoglobin required; $20\ \mathrm{g\cdot dl^{-1}}$ is the Hb concentration in packed cells and the volume to be transfused can then be calculated. For example, in a 4-kg infant with a Hb of $7\ \mathrm{g\cdot dl^{-1}}$ to be raised to $12\ \mathrm{g\cdot dl^{-1}}$:

$$12 - 7\ \mathrm{g\cdot dl^{-1}} = 5\mathrm{g\cdot dl^{-1}}\ \text{increase necessary}$$
$$\text{Blood volume } (80\ \mathrm{ml\cdot kg^{-1}} \times 4) = 320\ \mathrm{ml}$$
$$5\ \mathrm{g\cdot dl^{-1}} \times 320\ \mathrm{ml} = 16\ \mathrm{g\,Hb}$$
$$16\ \mathrm{g} \div 20\ \mathrm{g\cdot dl^{-1}} = 80\ \mathrm{ml\ packed\ cells\ required}$$

This can be transfused at a rate of 15 ml hourly.

Cross-matching

Blood as fresh as possible must be cross-matched for all major surgery and for operations where a blood loss of 10 per cent of the blood volume is anticipated. This includes most neonatal operations.

Haemorrhagic disorders

The cause of any haemorrhagic disorder in the newborn must be sought preoperatively and treated. The commonest cause of bleeding in the newborn is trauma during delivery. Bleeding due to coagulation defects is now uncommon since prophylactic treatment with vitamin K is routine.

Premature babies may have many deficiencies in clotting factors because of their immaturity. Sick neonates may develop disseminated intravascular coagulopathy (DIC) with a secondary platelet deficiency. The latter may also be caused by certain congenital infections such as rubella or primary bone marrow disease.

Haemorrhagic disease of the newborn is discussed on p. 25. DIC occurs in serious neonatal disease associated with hypotension, acid–base disturbances and severe sepsis. There is diffuse haemorrhage, and bleeding into the brain or lungs can cause death. A low platelet count is found together with deficiency of the consumed factors V, VII and fibrinogen together with degradation products of fibrinogen. Treatment with heparin may be successful, giving $1\ \mathrm{mg\cdot^{-1}}$ intravenously 4-hourly to keep the partial thromboplastin time below 100 seconds; this method is not so often used nowadays.

Initial screening tests must include a platelet count, prothrombin time and partial thromboplastin time, and treatment may involve the use of vitamin K, fresh-frozen plasma, fresh blood or plasma platelet concentrate. Administration of fresh platelet concentrate in a dose of $10\text{–}15\ \mathrm{ml\cdot kg^{-1}}$ provides all the necessary clotting factors as well as normally functioning platelets. If the platelets are normal, the same volume of fresh frozen plasma may be given. Most neonates tolerate such transfusions at 8–12-hourly intervals as they may be volume depleted by repeated haemorrhage.

Nervous system

Convulsions

Convulsions must be brought under control preoperatively. They are most frequent during the first 3 days of life, being related to birth asphyxia, trauma, intracranial haemorrhage, metabolic disorders such as hypoglycaemia and hypocalcaemia, and sepsis, particularly meningitis. The convulsions may vary from mild twitching to full grand mal seizures and coma.

The primary cause (e.g. hypocalcaemia or hypoglycaemia) must be sought and effectively treated. A severe seizure may prejudice the airway and increase the tissue oxygen demand, causing cyanosis; some form of artificial airway may therefore be necessary, as may an increased inspired oxygen concentration. The seizures must be controlled using either diazepam (Valium) by incremental intravenous injection of up to 1 mg·kg^{-1} body weight or phenobarbitone 2 mg·kg^{-1} 8-hourly or 5 per cent paraldehyde infusion 2 mg·kg^{-1} body weight over 2–3 hours. If there is evidence of raised intracranial pressure (bulging fontanelle), a trial of dexamethasone 0.5 mg·kg^{-1} is indicated. Neonatal meningitis, like all neonatal infections, must be treated promptly and effectively. Antibiotic therapy (involving gentamicin and ampicillin) is usually continued for 3 weeks.

Myasthenia

Neonatal myasthenia gravis is found in 10 per cent of babies born to mothers with this condition. The degrees of ptosis and of weakness correlate well with the anti-acetylcholine receptor titres present in the blood, the patient being an auto-immune phenomenon.

Fluid and electrolyte balance

Abnormal water and electrolyte metabolism

Abnormal water losses

Increased insensible water loss with prematurity, phototherapy and exposure to radiant heat has been mentioned on p. 33, as has increased urine volume in infants with water-losing renal disease. In the presence of excess water loss, either through the skin as in very low birth weight babies or infants under radiant heat canopies or through the bowel, the urine output will fall. If adequate fluid replacement is not given, plasma osmolarity may rise because of the limited ability of the neonatal kidney to concentrate the urine. On the other hand, when a high solute load is given, either intravenously or as unmodified cows milk, plasma hyperosmolarity may also occur because of the large amounts of urinary water required in which to excrete the solutes. The loss of saliva in patients with oesophageal atresia seldom causes much disturbance, but duodenal atresia may cause loss of gastric, duodenal, biliary and pancreatic secretions by vomiting. When obstruction occurs lower down the intestinal tract, both the volume and the complexity of the composition of lost fluid increase. In addition, lower intestinal obstructions are commonly associated with gross abdominal distension, which in turn causes increased capillary permeability and loss of crystalloid and colloid from the vessels in the bowel wall. As well as loss of alimentary secretions, intestinal obstruction is further complicated by starvation. It is reasonable to assume that the chemical composition of the neonate with congenital intestinal obstruction is normal at birth, but the fluid and electrolyte losses outlined above will become increasingly severe the longer diagnosis and treatment are delayed.

Sodium

Sodium loss usually leads to a loss in extracellular fluid volume, and this in turn may result in circulatory collapse, whereas pure water depletion tends to affect intracellular fluid volume, particularly in the brain. Similarly, sodium retention may lead to hypertension and oedema from expansion of extracellular fluid volume, whilst water retention causes the syndrome of water intoxication.

The concentration of sodium in the serum is determined by the relative amounts of sodium and water in the body. It is thus possible to have a normal serum sodium with severe salt depletion or overload if there are equivalent changes in body water. On the other hand, low serum sodium levels can occur with water overload even in the presence of normal body sodium. Sodium concentration in the serum of premature or term newborn infants is not significantly different from the normal adult range.

Potassium

Potassium concentrations above the normal adult range have been found on the first day of life by several workers. Potassium is the principal intracellular cation and may be lost from the body during starvation or injury in proportion to the loss of nitrogen. With renal or gastrointestinal loss of potassium, intracellular volume is maintained by sodium and hydrogen ions entering the cells. This causes a reduction in extracellular volume, intracellular acidosis and extracellular alkalosis. Impairment of potassium excretion as in advanced renal failure causes an increase in extracellular potassium concentration, with the risk of cardiac dysfunction. Cardiac arrhythmias commonly occur when serum potassium levels are low.

Principles of intravenous therapy

Intravenous fluid therapy is indicated only if absorption by the oral route is inadequate. Preoperative starvation should not exceed 4 hours; even in cases of intestinal atresia or obstruction, early diagnosis and treatment may prevent long periods of fluid deprivation. Bowel function usually returns fairly quickly after surgery in the neonate, and feeds of milk—preferably human—should be established as soon as possible, either orally or via a nasogastric or transanastomotic feeding tube.

Shock

In states of hypovolaemic shock, blood 20 ml·kg⁻¹ body weight, plasma or 5 per cent albumin should be infused rapidly, depending on the Hb and haematocrit. In severe cases, up to 40 ml·kg⁻¹ is needed. This is sometimes the case in states of severe peritonitis. Central venous pressure monitoring is useful in ensuring the optimum right atrial filling pressure.

As dehydration is corrected, the peripheral circulation will improve and core/periphery temperatures will approximate. Indeed, the state of the peripheral circulation is a very sensitive guide to cardiac output and filling pressures in the baby.

The aim in preparation for surgery must be to achieve an optimal clinical state, but there should be as little delay as possible in operating on babies with severe peritonitis or possible gangrenous bowel.

Deficit replacement (Table 2.1)

An infant who is clinically dehydrated has probably lost 50–100 ml·kg⁻¹ body weight (5–10 per cent). At 5 per cent dehydration there is loss of skin turgor, the fontanelles are slightly depressed and the baby is lethargic. At 10 per cent, the fontanelles and orbits are sunken, peripheral blood flow is poor and the body temperature may be high or low. Dehydration greater than 10 per cent affects the cardiovascular system and circulatory collapse is imminent.

If the deficit is severe, up to 20 ml·kg⁻¹ of physiological saline may be given, and its effect judged clinically (improved skin elasticity, reduced pulse rate, increased venous pressure and urine output). Children with water-losing renal disease may require 200 ml·kg⁻¹ per day or more, and their sodium intake should be increased to cover the abnormal losses. Intestinal losses should be replaced with physiological saline, though if a metabolic acidosis is present, some of the sodium may be administered as bicarbonate. It is not usually necessary to give more than 2 mmol·kg⁻¹ of sodium bicarbonate in the first instance unless acidosis is severe.

Sodium

Sodium deficits range from 0–4 mmol·kg⁻¹ in hypertonic dehydration to 8–12 mmol·kg⁻¹ in severe hypotonic dehydration. These should be replaced over a period of 6 hours, though more slowly in hypertonic states.

Hypertonic and hypotonic dehydration should be appropriately corrected, the former with 0.18 per cent saline because there is a total deficit of NaCl even though serum sodium may be as high as 180 mmol·l⁻¹. Care must be taken not to correct the deficiency too quickly or cerebral oedema will follow. Hypotonic dehydration is corrected with physiological saline. A high potassium (8 mmol·l⁻¹) should decrease with treatment of any associated

Table 2.1 Contents of commonly used intravenous fluids

Solution	Na$^+$ (mmol·l^{-1})	Cl$^-$ (mmol·l^{-1})	K$^+$ (mmol·l^{-1})	Ca^{2+} (mmol·l^{-1})	Lactate (mmol·l^{-1})	Cal·l^{-1}
0.9% Saline	154	154	—	—	—	—
0.45% Saline in 2.5% dextrose	77	77	—	—	—	95
0.18% Saline in 4% dextrose	31	31	—	—	—	150
Hartmann's solution	131	111	5.0	2.0	29	—
Half-strength Hartmann's solution	65.5	55.5	2.5	1.0	14.5	—
5% Dextrose	—	—	—	—	—	190

dehydration or acidosis. Indeed, a low total body potassium may be revealed after rehydration and supplements will then be necessary. Oral feeding should commence as soon as possible to minimize catabolic effects causing acidosis, ketosis and uraemia.

Hypernatraemia associated with dehydration should be treated slowly, using 5 per cent dextrose—possibly after initial correction of the hypovolaemia, using blood or plasma.

Treatment should be controlled by serum and urine electrolyte measurements. The osmolality ratio between plasma and urine should be 1 : 1.5. Normal serum osmolality is 285–310 $mOsm \cdot l^{-1}$ and urine approximately 450 $mOsm \cdot l^{-1}$. The amount of sodium required to restore the sodium content is largely related to the extracellular fluid volume, which is increased in the neonate to approximately 40 per cent of body weight. An amount equivalent to 20 per cent of body weight is commonly added to this to allow for intracellular requirements; this makes up the 'sodium space' of 0.6.

A useful formula for calculating the amount of sodium required to replace a deficit is:

Sodium required = deficit × body weight × 'sodium space'
(mmol)   (mmol$\cdot^{-1}$)   (kg)

A 3 kg neonate with a sodium deficit of 12 $mmol \cdot^{-1}$ would thus require $12 \times 3 \times 0.6 = 21.6$ mmol of sodium. Since physiological saline contains 154 $mmol \cdot l^{-1}$, this deficit would be corrected by infusion of $21.6/154 \times 1000$ ml = 140 ml physiological saline.

Potassium

Potassium deficit is more difficult to assess because the loss is mainly intracellular and only serum levels can be easily measured. The shift of potassium from the cells that occurs with the acidosis of birth and its return as the acidosis decreases have already been mentioned (p. 31). Similar shifts of potassium across the cell membrane occur with changes in acid–base state throughout life, and administration of bicarbonate will lead to a fall in plasma potassium.

Metabolic acidosis should be corrected using the formula:

Dose required (mmol) = base deficit × body weight (kg) × 0.3

It is usual to give half the calculated dose initially and then reassess the acid–base state.

Replacement of potassium deficit is not usually an urgent matter, though it may be in special circumstances such as open heart surgery. The concentration of potassium administered should not exceed 40 $mmol \cdot l^{-1}$ and not more than 5 $mmol \cdot kg^{-1}$ per day should be given. Adequate urine flow should be present (at least 1 $ml \cdot kg^{-1}$ per hour) and deficit replacement should be spread over several days.

Maintenance requirements

The intravenous requirement for maintenance of fluid balance for the full-term neonate on the first day of life is met by the administration of 20–40 ml·kg^{-1} body weight per day and increases by 20 ml·kg^{-1} per day until it reaches 120 ml·kg^{-1} per day towards the end of the first week. In very low birth weight babies (less than 1.5 kg) the maintenance fluid requirement at birth may be as much as double that at term, rising to 160 ml·kg^{-1} per day. Because it is easier to give too much intravenous fluid than too little, some authorities do not administer any fluid intravenously to full-term neonates in the first few days of life unless abnormal losses occur. It should be emphasized, however, that such losses almost always do occur in premature babies, mainly by insensible loss through the skin; in such babies the risks of hyperbilirubinaemia and hypoglycaemia can be minimized by infusion of appropriate quantities of 5 or 10 per cent dextrose.

Intraoperative fluid requirements should be based on the maturity of the baby, the length of preoperative fluid deprivation and an estimation of the fluid lost into body cavities. Any fluid given in the injection of diluted muscle relaxants or other drugs should be included in the overall fluid balance. The normal maintenance requirements should be reduced by approximately 30 per cent in the first 24 hours after major surgery because of the antidiuretic response to the stress of anaesthesia and surgery, though infants with abnormal kidneys may not show this response. Postoperative fluid regimens should, however, include appropriate replacement for gastrointestinal losses and increased insensible loss associated with prematurity or the use of overhead heating canopies. Maintenance requirements for sodium and potassium in the neonate are 3 mmol·kg^{-1} per 24 hours and 2 mmol·kg^{-1} per 24 hours, respectively, though sodium requirements are halved in the first week of life.

Potassium deficiency is not well reflected in measured serum levels; potassium should therefore be included in most solutions, though not at a rate exceeding 3 mmol·kg^{-1} in 24 hours. Potassium should be withheld in cases of renal failure.

Renal failure

The choice of treatment depends to a great extent on the primary cause; vigorous treatment of underlying conditions such as septicaemia, for example, must be undertaken at once. Control of water and electrolyte changes must be sought and the circulating blood volume restored by plasma or blood if the baby is anaemic.

Potassium levels over 9 mmol·l^{-1} will need treatment, and a temporary reduction may be achieved with a solution of insulin (0.5–1.0 units) and glucose (10–20 ml of 50 per cent) given intravenously. Dialysis may be necessary, and is indicated when the blood urea rises over 50 mmol·$^{-1}$ and there is persistent oliguria with less than 50 ml of urine per 24 hours and oedema following rehydration. Acidosis with the pH less than 7.25 and hyperkalaemia greater than 7.5 mmol·l^{-1} in spite of treatment are also indications for dialysis. Peritoneal dialysis is preferred, as complications are few and regimens are relatively simple.

Acidosis must be treated and monitored as described previously (p. 36). It is essential to maintain a normal pH if full benefit is to be obtained from any inotropic agents being administered.

Rapid deterioration in a vicious circle of falling cardiac output, hypotension, hypovolaemia, metabolic acidosis, hypoxia and further falls in cardiac output will occur unless the patient is treated vigorously. Terminal respiratory failure is a common sequel of renal failure in babies and is associated with their lower respiratory reserve.

Metabolism

Hypoglycaemia

Hypoglycaemia in the term baby is usually defined as $1.6 \, \text{mmol·l}^{-1}$ (30 mg per cent) or less, and in those of birth weights below 3 kg it is $1.1 \, \text{mmol·l}^{-1}$ (20 mg per cent) in the first 3 days of life. After this time the blood sugar should always be above $2.2 \, \text{mmol·l}^{-1}$ (40 mg per cent), and if found to be below this, it must be corrected. Unless the levels are very low, the hypoglycaemic baby may be asymptomatic though symptoms such as tremors, apnoea, cyanosis, apathy, hypotonia, hypothermia and convulsions are all described. The possibility of hypoglycaemia must be anticipated to prevent avoidable brain damage; 25–50 per cent of babies with symptomatic hypoglycaemia develop neurological sequelae. Babies very likely to become hypoglycaemic include premature and infants that are small for their maturity dates with poor deposits of fat and glycogen, infants of diabetic mothers and those asphyxiated at birth. Very premature infants born before fat and glycogen deposits have been laid down may become hypoglycaemic at any time during the first week or two of life, especially if they are severely ill or if their calorie intake is inadequate. In small-for-dates infants (less than 2.5 kg at term) the peak incidence of hypoglycaemia is usually found between 24 and 72 hours of age. At this stage glycogen stores have fallen whilst the infant, particularly if breast-fed, is still on a hypocaloric intake. There may be increased energy demands if the baby is nursed below the neutral temperature range. Infants of diabetic mothers have high insulin levels and may become hypoglycaemic within a few hours of birth. Since their homoeostatic mechanisms are usually working well, such an infant seldom comes to harm unless he is very ill or the mother was on sulphonylurea drugs. Infants with severe birth asphyxia may become hypoglycaemic shortly after resuscitation. Hypoglycaemia may, of course, be a symptom of some other condition such as glycogen storage disease or adenoma of the pancreas. By performing Dextrostix estimations and/or laboratory blood sugar determinations every 4–6 hours in the first 3 days of life for small-for-dates babies and others at risk, most cases of asymptomatic hypoglycaemia will be detected. If possible, early feeding should be undertaken, but where this is not possible an infusion of 10 per cent dextrose at a rate of 75–100 ml·kg⁻¹ per 24 hours should be set up. If the hypoglycaemia is unrelieved, the dextrose should be changed to 15 per cent. If more immediate correction is required, 1–2 ml·kg⁻¹ of 50 per cent dextrose should be given promptly. All intravenous fluids for infants should include dextrose. If the usual methods do not control the hypoglycaemia, steroids (prednisone 1 mg·kg⁻¹ 8-hourly) or ACTH (4 units 12-hourly) should be administered.

Hypocalcaemia

Hypocalcaemia is commonest in the first 2 days of life in sick babies. It is possibly due to immaturity of the parathyroid glands, though it may appear at 5–7 days in babies fed on cow's milk, which has a high phosphate content. Hypocalcaemia may develop during an exchange transfusion with acid–citrate–dextrose.

The signs of hypocalcaemia—which are mainly non-specific neurological signs such as irritability or failure to synchronize with a ventilator or, rarely, tetany or convulsions—are manifestations of a low ionized Ca^{2+} level, not necessarily fully reflected in total serum levels. The proportion which is protein bound can be estimated from the albumin level.

Treatment of hypocalcaemia is imperative and urgent if the total calcium level falls below 1.5 mmol·l⁻¹ or if the ionized calcium level falls below 0.7 mmol·l⁻¹. It is wise to treat ionized calcium levels below 0.95 mmol·l⁻¹. If convulsions occur, calcium should be given without waiting for the results of serum calcium estimations (1 ml·kg⁻¹ of 20 per cent calcium gluconate). In the absence of convulsions, hypocalcaemia should be treated by continuous infusion of a dilute (2 per cent) solution of calcium gluconate at a rate of 5 mg·kg⁻¹ per hour. Because calcium solutions are irritant, they should not be given into scalp veins, where tissue necrosis may occur. Calcium solutions are also incompatible with sodium bicarbonate.

Other metabolic disorders

Hypomagnesaemia may occur in association with hypocalcaemia, following exchange transfusion or following administration of diphenylhydantoin to the mother for the treatment of toxaemia of pregnancy. Treatment with 1 per cent magnesium sulphate intravenously should not exceed 5–10 ml at a rate of less than 1 ml per minute.

Inborn errors of metabolism occasionally require attention in the neonatal period. Galactosaemia may cause hypoglycaemia, and others such as hyperglycinaemia may cause acidosis. It is important to detect cases of phenylketonuria and maple syrup urine disease in order to take corrective measures to allow mental development to proceed normally.

Premedication

Atropine is the only commonly used premedicant drug for neonatal patients.

For infants weighing less than 2.5 kg, the dose is 0.15 mg; for those between 2.5 and 8 kg, the dose is 0.2 mg, by intramuscular injection 30–45 minutes preoperatively. This is the routine at the Hospital for Sick Children, London.

The antisialagogue action of atropine (and hyoscine) is less important nowadays since ether with its irritant effects on the tracheobronchial tree has largely been superseded, but its use remains more important in babies than in adults.

There is an increased risk of laryngeal spasm on extubation if the patient has excessive tracheobronchial secretions, and especially in those who have received halothane. Blockage of a narrow endotracheal tube with secretions is also a possibility. All babies who are to receive suxamethonium, cyclopropane or halothane should be given atropine as a vagolytic drug. Excessive drying of secretions is undesirable, especially in patients with cystic fibrosis or those suffering from dehydration, and in these a reduced dose may be used.

Hyoscine, which can cause excitation in the young, is not used in neonatal anaesthesia and its excessive drying action on the mucosa is probably undesirable. Some centres prefer the administration of atropine by intravenous injection during induction of anaesthesia to ensure immediate action, arguing that vagal tone tends to be low in newborn babies.

Competency of the cardio-oesophageal junction may be increased with atropine, which may be important in patients with gastric emptying problems such as pyloric stenosis, though a large nasogastric tube and gastric washouts should ensure full drainage of the stomach in all such patients.

Atropine has been incriminated in the production of febrile convulsions and, although there are other factors involved such as hypovolaemia, atropine is best avoided in the pyrexial or toxic patient, or a lower dose should be used. It can be administered intravenously if necessary.

No sedation is required for neonates preoperatively, though exceptionally it may be given to patients undergoing open heart surgery, which sometimes employs a technique of surface cooling. Babies are sensitive to all sedative drugs and their use must be limited to special circumstances. Morphine given to neonates in doses of one-third of the adult dose on a weight-for-weight basis reduces significantly the ventilatory response to carbon dioxide.

Vitamin K 1 mg intramuscularly should also be given because of its relative deficiency in the newborn and the immaturity of the liver enzyme system in synthesizing prothrombin.

References and further reading

Transport

Blake, A. M., McIntosh, N., Reynolds, E. O. R. and St Andrews, D. (1975). Transport of newborn infants for intensive care. *British Medical Journal* **4**, 13.

Hackel, A. (1975). A medical transport system for the neonate. *Anesthesiology* **43**, 258.

Preoperative assessment

Behrman, R. E. and Itsia, D. Y. Y. (1969). Summary of a symposium on phototherapy for hyperbilirubinemia. *Journal of Pediatrics* **75**, 718.

Bennett, E. J. (1975). *Fluids for Anesthesia and Surgery in the Newborn Infant.* Charles C. Thomas, Springfield, Illinois.

Bennett, E. J. (1975). Fluid balance in the newborn. *Anesthesiology* **43**, 210.

Brown, J. K. (1976). Fits in childhood. In: *A Textbook of Epilepsy.* Ed. by J. Laidlaw and A. Richens. Churchill Livingstone, Edinburgh and London.

Bush, G. H. (1971). Intravenous therapy in paediatrics. *Annals of the Royal College of Surgeons of England* **49**, 92.

Chessells, J. M. and Hardisty, R. M. (1974). Bleeding problems in the newborn infant. In: *Progress in Hemostasis and Thrombosis*, vol. II. Ed. by T. H. Spaet. Grune & Stratton, New York.

Cornblath, M. and Schwartz, R. (1976). *Disorders of Carbohydrate Metabolism in Infancy*, 2nd edn. Saunders, Philadelphia and Eastbourne.

Haworth, J. C. (1974). Neonatal hypoglycemia. How much does it damage the brain? *Pediatrics* **54**, 3.

Levin, S. E., Bakst, C. M. and Isserow, L. (1961). Sclerema neonatorum treated with corticosteroids. *British Medical Journal* **2**, 1533.

Lister, J. (1977). Surgical emergencies in the newborn. *British Journal of Anaesthesia* **49**, 43.

Rickham, P. P., Lister, J. and Irving, I. M. (eds) (1978). *Neonatal Surgery*, 2nd edn. Butterworths, London.

Roberton, N. R. C. (1979). Management of hyaline membrane disease. *Archives of Disease in Childhood* **54**, 838.

Schaffer, A. J. and Avery, M. E. (1977). *Diseases of the Newborn.* 4th edn. Saunders, Philadelphia and Eastbourne.

Scopes, J. W. (1977). Management of respiratory distress syndrome. *British Journal of Anaesthesia* **49**, 35.

Sinclair, J. C., Driscoll, J. M., Heird, W. C. and Winters, R. W. (1970). Supportive management of the sick neonate. *Pediatric Clinics of North America* **17**, 863.

Stanbury, J. B., Wyngaarden, J. B. and Fredrickson, D. S. (Eds) (1978). *The Metabolic Basis of Inherited Disease*, 4th edn. McGraw-Hill, New York and Maidenhead.

Swyer, P. R. (1975). *The Intensive Care of the Newly Born. Physiological principles and practice.* Monographs in Paediatrics, vol. 6. S. Karger, Basel; Wiley, Chichester.

Young, D. G. (1973). Fluid balance in paediatric surgery. *British Journal of Anaesthesia* **45**, 953.

Wilkinson, A. W. (1973). Some aspects of renal function in the newly born. *Journal of Pediatric Surgery* **8**, 103.

3

Anaesthesia—
basic principles

Anaesthetic equipment

Equipment necessary for paediatric anaesthesia must be specialized; adult apparatus is rarely, if ever, suitable for use in babies. Paediatric equipment must—especially if used with spontaneous breathing—have a low resistance to gas flow (less than $30\,cmH_2O\cdot l^{-1}$ per second during quiet breathing). It must be as light as possible without being cumbersome, should have minimal apparatus dead space (less than 5 ml) and include safety features to prevent kinking, obstruction or build-up of abnormal pressure within the airway. The work of breathing, which is higher in infancy anyway, will be increased by turbulent gas flow. Humidification and heating of inspired gases is desirable, as is scavenging of expired, polluting gases.

Circuits

For neonatal anaesthesia, the most commonly used circuit is the Ayre's T-piece, introduced in 1937. In 1950, Jackson Rees modified the basic T-piece, increasing the length of the expiratory limb and adding an open-ended reservoir bag (Fig. 3.1). Since then the circuit has been investigated extensively for controlled ventilation and spontaneous breathing in laboratory models and clinical anaesthesia for all age groups. With spontaneous ventilation there is no rebreathing if the fresh gas flow (FGF) is two and a half to three times the patient's minute volume. There is no dilution of the gases by air if the volume of the expiratory limb exceeds 75 per cent of the predicted tidal volume of the patient. The usual volume of the expiratory limb is 40 ml and that of the reservoir bag is 750 ml. The inspired gases can be warmed and humidified if required.

The T-piece fulfils the requirements for very low resistance, low dead space, convenience and simplicity, but its use of gases is wasteful and there is no reliable pressure-relief valve in the circuit. Scavenging of gases is most safely achieved by an *indirect* active system, as described on p. 87.

For controlled ventilation it is possible to reduce the fresh gas flow as some rebreathing may be an advantage, thus preventing the effects of inadvertent hyperventilation. In practice it is not advisable to reduce the flow below 4 litres per minute, as the bag becomes more difficult to use.

The Bain circuit, with coaxial tubing, has similar properties to the T-piece, and may be used as an alternative. Accidents have been reported

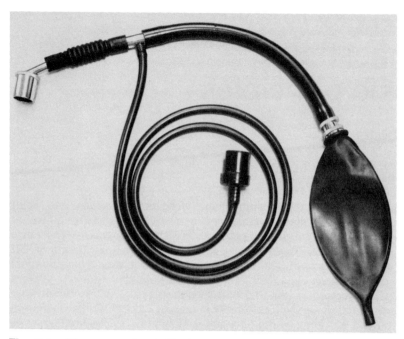

Fig. 3.1 The anaesthetic T-piece with face mask adaptor.

when the circuit has developed a malfunction and the fresh gas flows between the concentric tubing, as there is a massive increase in apparatus dead space. Scavenging of expired gases is easier with the Bain circuit (Fig. 3.2).

Circle absorption systems have been especially popular in the United

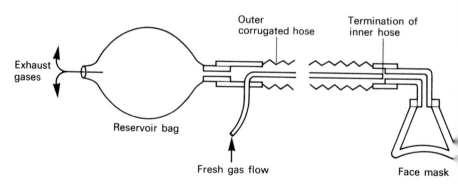

Fig. 3.2 Diagram of the Bain circuit for paediatric anaesthesia. (From Sumner, E. and Patrick, E. K. (1980).

States where light plastic tubing, gravity-operated silicone rubber valves, humidification, warming and scavenging are cited as advantages.

One-way valves are potentially dangerous in neonatal anaesthesia. They may stick and they introduce increased resistance and dead space into the circuit.

When controlled ventilation is required, as is usual in small babies, manual ventilation with the T-piece is the most satisfactory. If mechanical ventilation is necessary, machines are available (Sheffield or Amsterdam) which utilize a T-piece with an electronically timed mechanism to direct the FGF into the patient for a preset inspiratory time (Fig. 3.3). It is possible, however, to use other ventilators for neonatal anaesthesia.

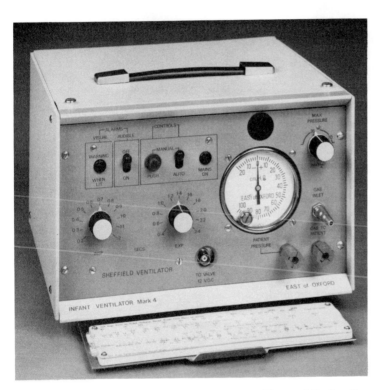

Fig. 3.3 The Sheffield infant ventilator (East of Oxford).

Face masks (Fig. 3.4)

Face masks are not used for long periods in small babies because general anaesthesia almost invariably involves intubation (p. 69). A good fit on the face is of equal or even greater importance than very low dead space, which in practice is reduced by streaming effects of the FGF within the mask. The Rendell-Baker mask has the lowest dead space, but may not make a good air seal on the baby's face. The Rendell-Baker divided airway further reduces dead space.

Airways

The commonly used airways in neonatal anaesthesia are the Phillips and the Guedel.

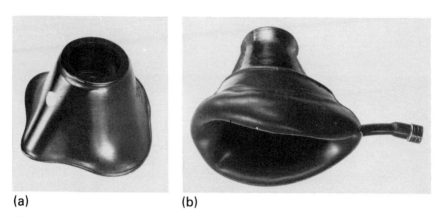

(a)   (b)

Fig. 3.4   Face masks suitable for neonatal use: (a) Rendell-Baker; (b) M & I E, with inflatable rim.

Laryngoscopes

Because of the anatomy of the infant's upper airway, a straight-bladed laryngoscope is more appropriate, and the glottis is usually viewed by lifting the epiglottis from its posterior surface. Suitable blades are the Anderson–Magill or Robertshaw (Figs. 3.5 and 3.6). The Anderson-Magill laryngoscope has the advantage of a hook on the handle with which the instrument may be stabilized on the index finger. If it is necessary to use intubating forceps as with nasotracheal intubation, the Robertshaw blade may be preferable. In the United States, the Wis-Hipple, Flagg or Miller blades are commonly used.

Endotracheal tubes

Plain endotracheal tubes of the Magill type are usually made of rubber or plastic; 3 mm inside diameter is usual for the term baby and 2.5 mm for the premature. The advantages of rubber include the possibility of reusage after autoclaving and easier insertion because of increased stiffness of the tube. It is claimed that there is a greater incidence of laryngeal spasm on extubation after using a red rubber tube, but for short-term use this is more likely to be related to incorrect timing of the extubation rather than to the material from

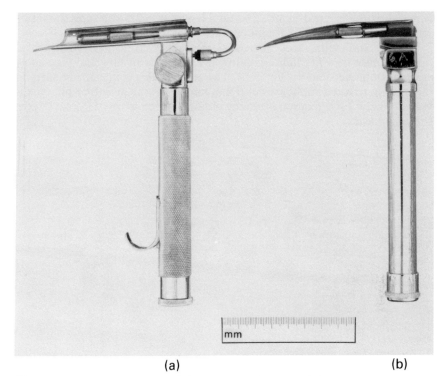

(a)   (b)

Fig. 3.5   Laryngoscopes: (a) Anderson-Magill; (b) Robertshaw.

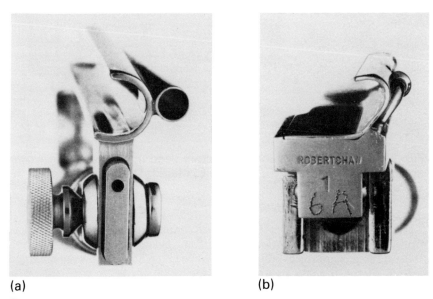

(a)   (b)

Fig. 3.6   Cross-sectional views of Fig. 3.5.

which the tube is constructed. The total length of a 2.5 mm tube should be 10 cm, and 12 cm for a 3.0 mm endotracheal tube.

Cardiff connectors are extremely satisfactory for small endotracheal tubes because they are light, with low resistance to air flow and they allow easy fixation and suction (Fig. 3.8). The angle of this connector imparts an ideal curve to a red rubber tube so that kinking in the mouth or pharynx is very unlikely. Firm fixation is readily obtained using strips of 2.5 cm stretch sticking plaster.

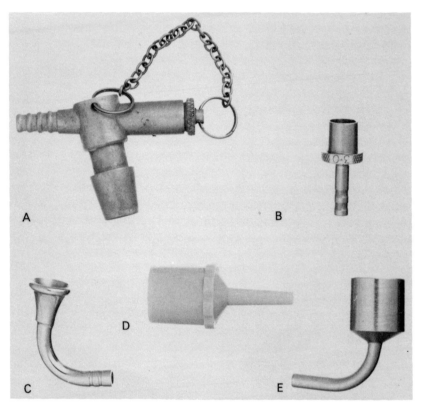

Fig. 3.7 Endotracheal tube connectors used in neonatal anaesthesia: A, Cardiff; B, Oxford; C, Magill; D, Portex 15 mm; E, Penlon, 15 mm.

Magill flexometallic tubes (Fig. 3.9) are commonly used for neurosurgical procedures, as kinking will not occur with any position of the head. Fixation of these tubes is not so easy and care must be taken not to allow the enlarged portion of the tube to pass between the vocal cords. A wire stilette is necessary to stiffen the tube for intubation. Firm fixation is particularly important for these endotracheal tubes in neurosurgical anaesthesia, where access may be difficult. Fixation involving strips of plaster around the tube sticking down over the neck and up over the cheeks is recommended.

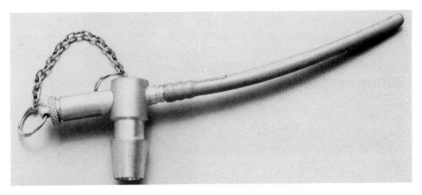

Fig. 3.8 Plain Magill tube with Cardiff connector.

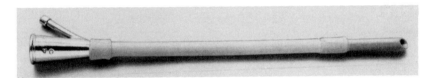

Fig. 3.9 Magill flexometallic tube.

Oxford tubes (Fig. 3.10) are used in anaesthesia for oesophagoscopy, some otolaryngological procedures and plastic surgery of the head and neck. The Oxford tube has an ideal shape to prevent inadvertent kinking in the pharynx and, thus, respiratory obstruction. A curved Magill connection is used and intubation is most satisfactorily carried out with a small, lubricated, gum-elastic bougie through the tube. This technique surmounts the difficulty occasionally experienced with Oxford tubes in a patient with an anterior larynx where the tip of the tube cannot be angled forwards to reach the glottis. These tubes have a tapered outside diameter so it is extremely important to use a tube of the correct size. If too large a tube is used, the larynx will be stretched as the tube is inserted, with subsequent oedema and stridor.

Cole pattern endotracheal tubes (Fig. 3.11) with a shouldered section are made of polyvinyl chloride, but the smallest sizes are unsatisfactory for spontaneous ventilation because of an unacceptably high resistance to breathing caused by turbulent air flow at the shoulder. The 8 French gauge (FG) size has an internal diameter of little more than 1 mm. They are unsuitable for prolonged intubation as fixation is not very firm and there is a tendency for the tube to move further into the trachea, thus dilating the glottis. If the

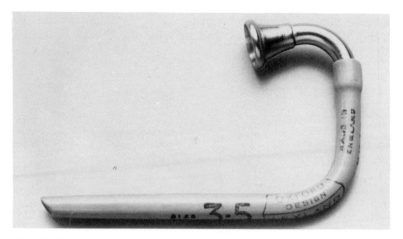

Fig. 3.10 Oxford tube with Magill curved connector.

shouldered part rests on the cricoid, the subglottic area will be damaged. Cases have been reported in which continued pressure by the oral tube has caused a cleft in the palate. Other cases have been reported in which accidental dislodgement of the tube has necessitated surgical removal from the oesophagus. However, these tubes are often used for neonatal resuscitation because they are easy for relatively inexperienced staff to use.

Anaesthetic apparatus should be sterilized between cases so that each patient has a clean circuit. Endotracheal tubes and connections are autoclaved and kept sterile until use. If a lubricant is used then this should also be sterile.

Apparatus concerned with intraoperative monitoring and temperature maintenance is discussed on p. 80 et seq.

Anatomy of the airway

The neonate has a relatively large head because of the advanced development of the brain, but the neck is short and the shoulders and chest are narrow.

Various anatomical differences can make the neonate difficult to intubate. The tongue is large in relation to the size of the oropharynx and this may interfere with visibility and the easy positioning of a laryngoscope blade.

The trachea is approximately 4 cm in length and between 6 and 8 mm in diameter in a term baby, and endobronchial intubation is more likely than in older children. The right main bronchus is more easily intubated than the left. The vocal cords lie opposite the lower border of the C4 vertebra and at about the fourth year of life are found at the adult level of C5 or C6. Thus,

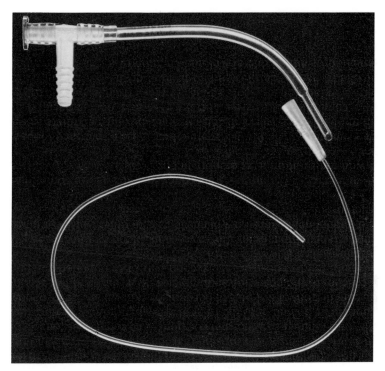

Fig. 3.11 Cole tube and suction catheter.

the infant glottis lies higher and more anteriorly than in the older child and is behind a soft and often 'folded' epiglottis. The infant epiglottis inclines to the posterior pharyngeal wall at an angle of 45 degrees, and the vocal cords are angled more forwards and downwards than in the adult. The anatomical differences mean that specialized equipment and techniques are required for intubation in this age group.

The narrowest part of a child's airway is at the level of the cricoid ring which is easily damaged by the inadvertent use of an endotracheal tube which is too large, but which may have passed through the glottis. Because there is a complete ring of cartilage at this level, any oedema will narrow the airway: 1 mm of mucosal oedema at the cricoid level may reduce the area of the airway by as much as 60 per cent in a newborn infant.

Basic techniques

Induction of anaesthesia and intubation

The baby is transferred to a prepared operating theatre from the surgical intensive care unit in a heated incubator providing neutral thermal environment. It is our practice to induce anaesthesia for neonates on the operating table prepared with a prewarmed electric heating pad and warm covering. The ambient temperature should be 25°C and the room draught-free. Higher temperatures are not recommended, as discomfort of the staff will then become a consideration.

The baby is removed from the incubator and at once placed on the operating table on the heating pad and swaddled in the warm coverings. Anaesthesia for neonates must involve intubation in the vast majority of cases, even for the most minor operations. The patency of the airway cannot be guaranteed with a face mask and spontaneous ventilation is rarely a part of neonatal anaesthesia. The respiratory system is so vulnerable to the depressant effects of inhalational anaesthesia and reduction in functional residual capacity (FRC) that controlled ventilation should be an integral part of the anaesthetic technique. This is only possible using an endotracheal tube because the compliance of the chest is lower than that of the abdomen and abdominal distension would tend to occur if assisted ventilation with a face mask were attempted.

In the newborn, endotracheal intubation is most commonly performed before induction of anaesthesia, but after a minute or two of preoxygenation from a face mask. The manoeuvre is easily performed without trauma even in vigorous babies because they have relatively little muscular strength. If the airway is secured before anaesthesia, there is less risk of aspiration of regurgitated gastric contents into the lungs. Moreover, if intubation difficulties are encountered (such as the small larynx sometimes associated with tracheo-oesophageal fistula, subglottic stenosis, laryngeal webs or other congenital airway problems), there is less difficulty in maintaining full oxygenation of the infant while a smaller endotracheal tube is selected. On the other hand, there may be great difficulty in maintaining an airway with a mask after induction of anaesthesia in the newborn and the risk of regurgitation is increased, especially if slight respiratory obstruction occurs. Laryngeal spasm is also a possibility.

After preoxygenation to help protect the infant from hypoxaemia during the breath-holding associated with awake intubation, laryngoscopy is performed. Correct holding of the baby is essential for easy intubation (Fig. 3.12)..The head should not be extended at the neck, but at the atlanto-occipital joint, producing a 'sniffing' position. The arms are restrained within the warm covers and the assistant presses the baby's shoulders firmly onto the surface of the operating table with both his palms while his fingers hold the head steadily on either side. The position of the head is crucial for successful intubation. The shoulders must not be allowed to rise from the table. The anatomy of the infant larynx is such that the best view is usually obtained using a straight-bladed laryngoscope, the tip of which picks up the epiglottis from its posterior surface; however, if the epiglottis is very short, the best view of the larynx may be obtained with the tip of the blade in the vallecula (Fig. 3.13).

The mouth is opened with the index finger of the right hand, the laryngoscope blade put into it from the right to keep the tongue over to the left, and advanced into the pharynx beyond the glottis. It is then withdrawn until the

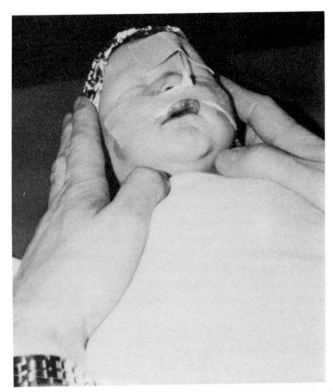

Fig. 3.12 Intubation, 1. Correct way to hold the baby.

glottis is visualized and the vocal cords are seen moving as the baby takes a breath. If an Anderson–Magill blade is used, the hook should rest on the left index finger and the left little finger can then press the larynx back to improve the view. A plain Magill tube of rubber (autoclaved) or plastic (disposable) is gently inserted into the trachea as the baby takes an inspiratory breath. If firm resistance is met, a smaller tube should be used. Most neonates require a 3.0 mm or 2.5 mm (inside diameter) endotracheal tube. The correct sized tube is that which is easily inserted and which has a small air leak around it, and is thus not too tight at the cricoid ring. This should be tested by light distension of the lungs with the T-piece bag, when an air leak should be audible. A tube which is too tight may damage the mucosa at the cricoid and cause postoperative oedema and stridor. Ulceration of the mucosa may progress to subglottic stenosis. After auscultation of the chest to confirm that the tip of the tube has not passed into one or other main bronchus, it is firmly secured with strips of 2.5 cm wide stretch sticking plaster. An infant airway is inserted into the mouth alongside the endotracheal tube to splint it and prevent it from kinking. If an oesophageal stethoscope and/or a nasogastric tube are required, these are more easily placed before an oral airway is inserted.

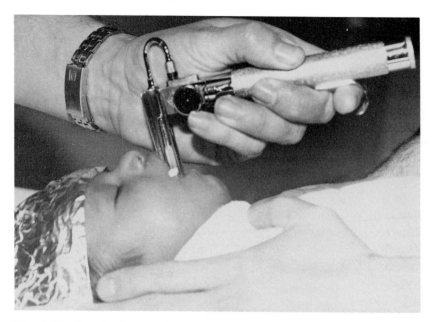

Fig. 3.13 Intubation, 2. Correct way to hold the laryngoscope.

Nasal endotracheal intubation is rarely used in the operating theatre except in cases already receiving respiratory support or for whom respiratory support is planned postoperatively. The technique is very well established indeed for prolonged airway management, but is technically more difficult to perform in the awake neonate because of the need for instrumentation in the mouth with intubating forceps. It is therefore safer to undertake oral intubation first and change to nasal intubation later if required.

Awake intubation should be attempted in all babies under 21 days of life, as the ease of the intubation is related to the muscular resistance rather than to the age of the baby. If the baby is very vigorous and the muscular resistance great, attempts at awake intubation should be abandoned and anaesthesia induced using the technique with which the anaesthetist is most familiar; for example, inhalational induction with oxygen/nitrous oxide/halothane; cyclopropane/oxygen (1 litre of each per minute) or intravenous induction with thiopentone 2—4 mg·kg^{-1} body weight. Induction of anaesthesia is followed by the administration of a muscle relaxant—commonly suxamethonium 1 mg·kg^{-1} intravenously.

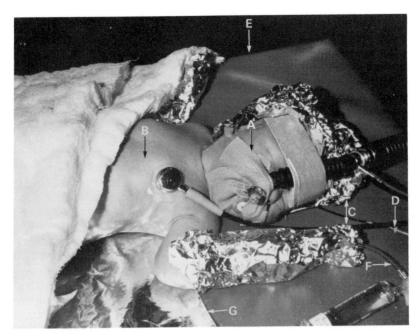

Fig. 3.14 The anaesthetized neonate prepared for surgery, showing: A, fixation of endotracheal tube; B, precordial stethoscope; C, foil; D, thermistor; E, heating pad; F, intravenous line; and G, dry diathermy plate.

The difficult intubation

The neonate may be more difficult to intubate than an adult or an older child because of the anatomical differences already described. In addition, there are certain conditions which may cause further difficulty: where there is immobility of the cervical spine, as in Klippel–Feil syndrome, micrognathia with Pierre Robin syndrome, or macroglossia with Hurler's syndrome, laryngoscopy may be very awkward or even impossible. The presence of a cleft palate and an anteriorly placed premaxilla will hinder easy intubation and the blade of the laryngoscope may slip into the cleft. Babies with conditions such as cystic hygroma and haemangiomata of the head and neck with respiratory obstruction may also be very difficult to intubate.

In these situations awake intubation should be performed where possible, but if anaesthesia is necessary for an older neonate, only inhalational techniques are advisable. Success is best achieved with care and patience. A selection of sterile endotracheal tubes down to 2.5 mm internal diameter should always be available. If a 2.5 mm tube will not pass into the trachea, the smallest Cole pattern tube may be required. A choice of straight- and curved-bladed infant laryngoscopes should be available and also a fairly stiff gum elastic bougie. Laryngoscopy should be performed after preoxygenation; if visualization of the glottis is difficult, its whereabouts can be deduced by seeing bubbles of saliva as the baby breathes in and out. It may be possible to bring the glottis into view by pressing on the front of the neck. In particularly difficult cases it may help to thread the gum elastic bougie through the endotracheal tube and allow it to emerge by 2 cm or so at the tracheal end. The tip of the bougie can then be bent anteriorly and used to guide the tube into the trachea. Occasionally, it may be necessary to use the bougie alone to find the glottic opening. The chosen endotracheal tube is then threaded over the bougie into the trachea. If the endotracheal tube connector is curved, this is better inserted after the tube is in the trachea and the bougie has been removed.

The same techniques are also used when inhalational anaesthesia is necessary. Respiratory obstruction occurring after induction may be relieved by turning the baby on its side or even prone. Early insertion of an oral airway is less likely to provoke coughing and laryngeal spasm in this age group than in the older child. A nasopharyngeal airway is an alternative, though it carries the risk of an epistaxis. When the baby is sufficiently deeply anaesthetized (usually with oxygen and halothane), laryngoscopy and intubation are performed as described above. Muscle relaxants must not be used at this stage, as valuable evidence of the whereabouts of the glottis revealed by respiratory movements will be lost. Muscle relaxants must not be used in any case of respiratory obstruction until it has been proved possible to ventilate the lungs with a face mask. Inhalational induction of anaesthesia, especially in the presence of respiratory obstruction, may be aided by the application of some constant distending pressure on the lungs. This is achieved by maintaining a taut anaesthetic T-piece reservoir bag.

Intravenous cannulation

Intravenous access is mandatory for general anaesthesia in neonatal patients. Suitable veins may be found on the dorsum of the hand or at the wrist, on the feet or the scalp. Metal scalp vein needles are not satisfactory for prolonged use because they tend to cut out of the vein, though they may be easier to insert successfully; 20 gauge and 22 gauge cannulae are available manufactured in polypropylene (Medicut) or Teflon (Abbocath, Jelco or Venflon). Teflon is less thrombogenic, but is softer than polypropylene so is more likely to kink unless fixation is meticulous and the arm or leg is securely splinted. Correct holding of the limb is essential for successful venepuncture. If the wrist is squeezed too tightly, blood flow will be interrupted and the veins will collapse; if held too loosely, venous distension will not be achieved. The assistant holding the wrist must also slightly stretch the skin of the hand. After cleansing the skin with spirit, a hole beside the vein is made with a lancet. This is always necessary because, otherwise, Teflon cannulae buckle over the needle as they are advanced through intact skin.

Some anaesthetists prefer to perform the manoeuvre single-handed and distend the vein by squeezing the wrist (or ankle) between the index and middle fingers of the left hand. Optimal venous distension and stretching of the overlying skin are achieved more easily in this way.

After successful venepuncture and careful fixation of the cannula, a three-way stopcock is fitted and the wrist (or foot) secured with a small arm splint. Intravenous fluids are usually given by means of a constant infusion pump, though these are strictly necessary only for intravenous alimentation or for the administration of inotropic agents. Care must be taken to watch for signs of extravasation around the vein when an infusion pump is used. A giving set incorporating a microburette is a suitable alternative, though it is a wise precaution to fill the chamber only with the requirements for 1 hour at a time.

Blood or plasma is required when the estimated blood loss has reached 10 per cent of the calculated blood volume (see p. 24). It is usual to transfuse with plasma (plasma protein fraction) up to 20 per cent of the blood volume if the haematocrit is over 45 per cent and the Hb over 15 $g \cdot dl^{-1}$. Blood should be as fresh as possible and in small packs to avoid waste. The blood may be administered through a standard giving set but is given by syringe, using a three-way tap for accuracy. Microfilters are not used routinely but are indicated where massive transfusion is expected or if the patient has pulmonary vascular disease. Standard warming coils are not used routinely, but some attempt must be made to raise the blood temperature from the storage level. Adequate warming of the blood is achieved if the standard tubing of the giving set is held in a thermostatically controlled water bath and blood drawn slowly through the tubing into the syringe.

Neuromuscular blocking agents

There is still controversy concerning the effects of the muscle relaxants on newborn babies. There are many reports of the sensitivity of the neonatal neuromuscular junction to tubocurarine and relative resistance to suxamethonium—the so-called 'myasthenic response'. It is generally agreed that some form of sensitivity to non-depolarizers does exist in the newborn for the first 7 days of life, though there is a wide variation in response. *In vitro* experiments show that increased sensitivity of the neonatal neuromuscular junction to these relaxants stems from its immaturity. At birth the muscle fibres are sensitive to acetylcholine throughout their length; only after a few weeks does the normal adult end-plate sensitivity develop, and then only if the innervation to the muscle is normal. At the same time that reduction of the sensitive area of the neuromuscular junction occurs, there are changes in the frequency and amplitude of the miniature end-plate potentials. These are greater in amplitude but less frequent in the neonate than the adult. These changes seem to correspond with the change in sensitivity to tubocurarine. The effective dose of tubocurarine to produce a 90 per cent block of thumb adduction in response to supramaximal single shock nerve stimulation has been shown to be 0.34 $mg \cdot kg^{-1}$ body weight in infants under 10 days of age—the same as infants of other age groups. What is different in the very young group is the wide variation in response, though all recovery times are comparable. Such differences in response could be related to the large extracellular fluid volume of the newly born and to the variability in size of this fluid compartment in which the drug is distributed. Evidence does seem to rule out quantitative changes in plasma protein concentration and, thus, bioavailability of the drug as a cause of the increased sensitivity of newborn babies to the non-depolarizers, but it does not necessarily preclude qualitative changes in binding to plasma proteins. One experimental series (Bennett *et al.*, 1976) showed that it is necessary to give an initial bolus injection for curarization of 0.25 mg·kg^{-1} tubocurarine in the first 7 days of life, 0.4 mg·kg^{-1} from days 7 to 14 and 0.5 mg·kg^{-1} thereafter. However, neonatal sensitivity has also been found to pancuronium compared with tubocurarine. At birth, pancuronium is nine times as potent as tubocurarine, though this drops to six times by 28 days of life. Because of this, pancuronium doses of 0.04 mg·kg^{-1} are safest in babies of less than 7 days old, though after this 0.06 mg·kg^{-1} may be used. After the first 2 weeks of life, infants require similar doses to adults on a weight-for-weight basis (Fig. 3.15).

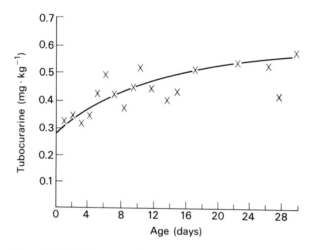

Fig. 3.15 Tubocurarine requirement during the neonatal period. (After data of Bush and Stead, 1962)

It seems that the development of normal adult response to tubocurarine is related more to the postnatal age than to the gestational age, and perhaps it is the greater neuromuscular activity after birth which stimulates the development of the mature end-plate characteristics.

Whether increased sensitivity to tubocurarine results from immaturity of the neuromuscular junction, differences in dilution of the drug or its binding by plasma proteins does not alter the need for careful titration of the drug dose against the response. Indeed the possibility of wide variations in patients less than 1 week old makes such a titration mandatory. Particular care must be taken in the premature, if the patient is acidotic or hypothermic in the presence of certain of the antibiotics (amikacin and gentamicin) and anaesthetic agents such as halothane. Tubocurarine in clinical doses has little cardiovascular effect in the newborn.

The effects of suxamethonium in the neonate are probably no different from those in the adult; reports of a decreased sensitivity may relate to the larger extracellular fluid volume throughout which the drug is distributed, in spite of lower plasma cholinesterase activity in infants up to 6 months of age. It is suggested that there is an increased tendency for the newborn to develop a prolonged action of suxamethonium (phase II block) and doses in excess of $5\,mg\cdot kg^{-1}$ should be avoided. However, phase II block in neonates has seldom been reported in clinical practice.

Both tubocurarine and suxamethonium must be given incrementally and the effects of each dose carefully assessed before more is given. Either drug is then extremely satisfactory and both have been used in neonatal anaesthesia for many years with great safety.

Tubocurarine should be diluted to a concentration of $0.5\,mg\cdot ml^{-1}$ and after intubation 0.5 mg may be given intravenously. Premature babies should receive 0.25 mg. Increments of 0.25 mg (0.125 mg in prematures) may be given to gain control of the ventilation, without exceeding a total dose of 1 mg for the full-term newborn. It is our practice to supplement anàesthesia with low concentrations of halothane (0.25–0.5 per cent) at the start of an operation, to avoid, where possible, the need for higher doses of relaxants. This should be discontinued at least 20 minutes before the end of the operation. Increments of tubocurarine may be given intraoperatively when necessary, in doses one-tenth of the original total dose. No such dose should be given within 20 minutes of the end of the operation.

The initial dose of pancuronium should be 0.1 mg with increments of 0.05 or 0.025 mg to achieve the desired control of ventilation.

Suxamethonium is diluted to a concentration of $2.5\,mg\cdot ml^{-1}$ and increments of 2.5 mg are given intravenously as necessary. The degree of muscular relaxation is best judged clinically from the abdominal musculature and the muscle tone in the fingers. An intermittent suxamethonium technique may be used for any neonatal operation (other than cardiac), but is probably better reserved for shorter operations to avoid the possibility of a phase II block. Again, it is our practice to supplement anaesthesia with low concentrations of halothane (0.25–0.5 per cent) for short periods of time during controlled ventilation in such cases, but to discontinue it well before the end of surgery.

At least 20–30 minutes must elapse between the last dose of tubocurarine and the end of the operation if full reversal is to be achieved easily. A mixture of atropine ($0.025\,mg\cdot kg^{-1}$) and neostigmine ($0.05\,mg\cdot kg^{-1}$) is given intravenously, from the same syringe, for reversal of residual curarization.

Inadequate reversal, as judged by poor respiratory effort, poor muscle tone, tracheal tug, intercostal recession and possibly raised $P\mathrm{aco_2}$, may be caused by a variety of factors. There may have been actual overdose or the administration of an increment of drug too near the end of the operation. The dose may be relatively too large because the effect of the drug has been potentiated by other agents, commonly halothane. Poor reversal will be seen in acidotic, hypothermic, hypoglycaemic babies and if the ionized calcium level is low. The last has a role in release of acetylcholine in the neuromuscular junction, and if low levels are suspected, 10 per cent calcium gluconate 15 mg·kg^{-1} should be given by slow intravenous injection.

Maintenance of anaesthesia

Controlled ventilation is the technique of choice, as respiratory depression easily occurs with spontaneous ventilation. After intubation it is our practice to induce light general anaesthesia with a 50 per cent oxygen/50 per cent nitrous oxide mixture and up to 0.5 per cent halothane with gentle assisted ventilation while an intravenous cannula and temperature monitoring probes are inserted and ECG electrodes are applied. It is possible that a high Pao_2 during the short duration of anaesthesia in a very low birth weight infant might cause retrolental fibroplasia, and the Pao_2 should be monitored during anaesthesia in such infants. As soon as venous access is established, carefully titrated doses of relaxant are given as previously described. Arterial and central venous cannulation are undertaken at this stage if necessary.

The closing volume in the neonatal lung is greater than the functional residual capacity, so airway closure occurs within normal tidal respiration. Controlled ventilation ensures that adequate alveolar ventilation is taking place and some positive end-expiratory pressure (PEEP) helps to maintain an adequate residual lung volume. Most paediatric anaesthetists feel it is safer to ventilate neonates by hand, rather than with a mechanical ventilator, except in special circumstances such as cardiac surgery. A ventilatory rate of 30–40 is employed (slower than the infant would be breathing spontaneously) with pressures of 25–30 cmH$_2$O and a fresh gas flow of 4 litres. It is usual to obtain a PEEP of about 5 cmH$_2$O during manual ventilation thus helping to preserve the FRC.

Inspired gases for neonatal anaesthesia should reach the patient fully humidified at a temperature not less than 33°C. This prevents damage to the mucosal lining of the respiratory tract by dry gases and therefore helps preserve mucociliary function and, possibly more important, minimizes heat loss from the baby. Certainly such gases, fully saturated at body temperature, will influence the thermal balance but there is an increased risk of infection from the humidifiers.

The aim is to produce mild hyperventilation—a safe procedure unless the patient is hypovolaemic from dehydration or haemorrhage. Great care must be taken with controlled ventilation in the presence of lung cysts because of the risk of tension pneumothorax, or with tracheo-oesophageal fistula because of gastric distension. Controlled ventilation is *not* contraindicated in these conditions, but extra vigilance is required and only gentle ventilation employed. For those unused to ventilating newborn babies by hand, a manometer may be incorporated in the T-piece circuit so that the actual pressures applied can be seen. Manual ventilation is the preferred technique for neonatal anaesthesia because minute-to-minute changes in compliance can be detected. This is especially important in thoracic surgery. Mechanical ventilators employing an electronic timing device to occlude the expiratory limb of a T-piece do exist (such as the Sheffield or Amsterdam) but are not used for neonates as a rule.

While every attempt should be made to provide adequate anaesthesia for the neonate undergoing surgery, it must be stressed that excessive doses of inhalational agents are dangerously depressing to the cardiovascular, respiratory and central nervous systems.

Halothane is an ideal agent for use in children, even for repeated anaesthesia, as the adult problem of possible hepatic sensitization to this agent does not seem to arise. The level of anaesthesia is rapidly controlled and at low doses has very little depressant effect on the cardiovascular system, except in patients with cardiac failure. The minimum alveolar concentration (MAC) is 1.1 for neonates (0.75 for adults).

Induction with halothane takes longer in a neonate than in an older child because of its high effective dead space/tidal volume ratio (50 per cent) and its increased physiological right-to-left shunt caused by the encroachment of the closing volume into tidal breathing.

Maintenance with intermittent halothane 0.25–0.5 per cent with 50 per cent oxygen 50 per cent nitrous oxide gives excellent anaesthetic results, allowing lower doses of relaxants. If the halothane is discontinued 20 minutes before the end of the operation, the patient should be fully awake after reversal of the relaxant.

Enflurane does not seem to have any particular advantages over halothane in this age group.

Intravenous analgesics have no place in neonatal anaesthesia except for those patients to be mechanically ventilated postoperatively such as after cardiac surgery.

Older, vigorous neonates undergoing short operations such as herniotomy may be allowed to breathe spontaneously a mixture of nitrous oxide, oxygen and halothane, though this is not recommended as a general rule. Anaesthesia for bronchoscopy also requires spontaneous ventilation in most cases (p. 140).

After the surgical procedure has finished and atropine and neostigmine have been given (in a dose of atropine 0.025 mg·kg^{-1} and neostigmine 0.05 mg·kg^{-1}), controlled ventilation continues with 100 per cent O_2, perhaps including 2–5 per cent CO_2, until full spontaneous ventilation has been re-established. The baby is covered with fresh, warmed wrappings. Suction through the endotracheal tube may be carried out using a fine sterile suction catheter if secretions are present, though not as a routine. As neonates are obligatory nose breathers, careful suctioning of the nostrils is done, using a soft rubber suction catheter.

Extubation

Extubation is carried out when the baby is *fully awake* (moving all limbs, eyes open) and respiratory effort is judged to be fully adequate in terms of depth, rate and absence of signs of distress such as intercostal recession and nasal flaring. The tube is withdrawn during compression of the T-piece reservoir bag so that the infant coughs the moment the tube leaves the trachea. The practice of extubating with a suction catheter down the tube is to be condemned because serious hypoxaemia may occur and there is a risk of aspiration of pharyngeal contents into the lungs as the first respiratory movement is inspiration.

There are many factors involved in poor respiratory function postoperatively, including pulmonary dysfunction such as hypoplasia occurring with diaphragmatic hernia or aspiration in tracheo-oesophageal fistula (see Chapter 4). Of the anaesthetic causes of postoperative respiratory insufficiency, inadequate reversal of the relaxant should be considered first. The dose of relaxant may be excessive or increments may have been given too late, but the effects of normal doses are intensified in the presence of high concentrations of inhalational anaesthetics or diazepam transferred via the placenta from the mother. Reversal difficulties may be experienced if the patient is hypothermic, acidotic, low in ionized Ca^{2+}, very premature or has a low cardiac output. Such patients may need a period of mechanical ventilation while these abnormalities are corrected. Hypoventilation leads to pulmonary atelectasis, hypoxia, acidosis and circulatory failure.

After careful assessment, the baby is returned to its heated incubator for the journey back to the intensive care unit.

Patient care during anaesthesia

Careful and continuous monitoring of the clinical status of the patient is essential during any anaesthetic. Because of the high metabolic rate and reduced respiratory reserve of the neonate, the clinical condition can deteriorate very rapidly and no piece of apparatus has yet been designed which will replace the meticulously careful well-trained clinical anaesthetist. There are, however, several devices available which help in patient monitoring, and the best of these are those which make the contact between the anaesthetist and the patient closer rather than more remote. In addition, a number of pieces of monitoring equipment are available which can give the anaesthetist information which cannot be obtained by direct clinical observation. It is also important to monitor not only the patient's well-being but also the function of the increasingly complicated pieces of anaesthetic equipment appearing in operating theatres.

Monitoring equipment must be reliable and easy to use, and should not by its size or design adversely affect the characteristics of the anaesthetic circuit or interfere with the safe conduct of the anaesthetic. Alarms should be fitted where appropriate, though these may fail or be set off by artefacts. Unnecessary bleeps and noises can be distracting both to the surgeon and anaesthetist.

Respiration

In the spontaneously breathing patient, monitoring of the airway and adequacy of respiration is carried out by observation of the movements of the reservoir bag of the anaesthetic T-piece. Almost all neonatal anaesthesia is carried out using controlled ventilation, however, and in this case the movements of the chest wall must be continuously watched. When manual ventilation is used, the anaesthetist can sense changes in compliance and resistance of the respiratory system or obstruction of the airway by changes in the 'feel' of the reservoir bag of the anaesthetic circuit with each breath. When mechanical ventilation is used, such changes are reflected by changes in the airway pressure dial of the ventilator, though these are less easily detected. The use of a precordial stethoscope is also helpful in monitoring inflation of the lungs, but can only be used as a continuous monitor for long periods of time if employed in conjunction with a monoaural earpiece. A Wright's respirometer or similar respiration meter may be used on the expiratory port of a mechanical ventilator, and on some ventilators respiration is monitored by the incorporation of one or more pneumotachographs.

Gross changes in oxygenation can be easily detected clinically, but changes in carbon dioxide tension cannot; if an absolute assessment of blood gas status is required, arterial blood gas analysis is performed. The problems of blood gas measurements in the newborn are described on p. 151. In practice, arterial lines are only used in neonatal anaesthesia for major surgery, particularly cardiac surgery. It may be difficult to obtain an arterial sample quickly in the operating theatre if an indwelling arterial line is not in place, and if a central venous pressure line is available a sample from this may be helpful. Serious arterial hypoxaemia is unlikely to be present if the oxygen tension in this central venous sample is above 5.3 kPa (40 mmHg). The measurement of cutaneous oxygen and carbon dioxide tensions has also been mentioned on p. 152, but the usefulness of this technique in the operating theatre is limited at least in short operations by the fact that the electrode takes about 15 minutes to stabilize. Some electrodes are adversely affected by anaesthetic gases. Monitoring of cutaneous oxygen tension may be helpful, however, during anaesthesia in premature neonates, where the risk of retrolental fibroplasia is high because the retinal vessels are susceptible to the effects of high arterial oxygen tensions. In these cases, the inspired oxygen concentration should also be measured, and the arterial oxygen tension in the upper limb arteries should be kept between 6.7 and 10.7 kPa (50–80 mmHg).

Heart and circulation

It is more difficult to assess cardiovascular status clinically during anaesthesia than to assess respiration, though useful information can be obtained by careful observation of the peripheral circulation and by keeping a finger on the axillary or femoral pulse. The following apparatus is therefore frequently used in addition.

Precordial stethoscope

The precordial stethoscope (Fig. 3.16) provides useful information about the heart sounds and heart rate, and reduction in intensity of the heart sounds may indicate a fall in blood pressure or cardiac output. The chest piece should be sufficiently small to sit comfortably on the neonatal chest and should be securely fixed. The smallest available oesophageal stethoscope (12 FG) is sometimes too large to be used in the neonate, though it can be very useful especially when there is difficult access to the chest.

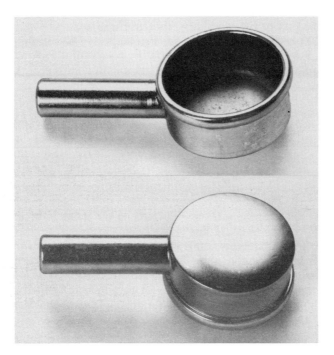

Fig. 3.16   The chest piece of a precordial stethoscope.

Blood pressure

Blood pressure measurement has been made easier in the newborn with the development of Doppler ultrasonic flowmeters. The conventional method of auscultation of the Korotkoff sounds is unsatisfactory in the operating theatre due to difficulty of access, though an electronic device is available which uses this technique with a microphone placed under the cuff. The signals from the microphone are amplified so that an audible or visual display of systolic and diastolic blood pressures can be produced. Blood pressure can also be estimated from the oscillations produced in an aneroid gauge as the cuff deflates, by palpation of the radial pulse or by the technique of oscillotonometry.

The ultrasonic measurement of blood pressure depends on the use of an occlusive cuff and an ultrasonic transducer placed over the brachial or radial artery. The transducer consists of an ultrasonic signal generator and a receiver. The change in frequency associated with blood flow in the artery is used to record systolic and diastolic blood pressures. The output from the transducer is amplified and filtered, and may be used to produce an audible signal or a printed record.

Whichever system of measurement of blood pressure is used, the cuff should be wide enought to cover two-thirds of the upper arm. In practice, this means that a cuff width of 4 cm is required for neonates.

Intra-arterial blood pressure monitoring is preferable when continuous monitoring is necessary or when arterial blood samples are required. In the newborn this can be obtained by catheterization of the umbilical artery. A size 5 FG polythene cannula is inserted in infants weighing over 1.5 kg or size 3½ FG for infants weighing less than 1.5 kg. Cannulae should be radio-opaque, and the tip of the cannula should be passed into the descending aorta below the origin of the inferior mesenteric and renal arteries at the level of the L2 vertebra. In the older neonate the radial artery can often be cannulated percutaneously using a 22 standard wire gauge (s.w.g.) polythene or Teflon cannula. This should be connected to a pressure trans-ducer by means of a short length of narrow-bore tubing and a three-way stopcock. Continuous flushing by means of a slow infusion pump using small volumes of heparinized dextrose or dextrose saline (1000 units of heparin per litre of fluid) minimizes the risk of thrombus formation and cannula blockage. Care must be taken to avoid the inadvertent injection of drugs into the artery. If the artery cannot be cannulated percutaneously, it may be necessary to expose it surgically and insert a similar cannula under direct vision. Although arterial cannulation is often followed by a temporary period of obstruction to blood flow, the incidence of long-term serious complications of radial and brachial artery cannulation in infants is very low.

Electrocardiogram

The ECG is a good monitor of pulse rate and disturbances of rhythm, though it provides no information about blood pressure or cardiac output. ECG recorders suitable for use in operating theatres should have a high common mode rejection ratio and therefore suppress unwanted signals from other pieces of electrical apparatus. It is useful to have an easily read trace, a rate counter and a freeze capacity on the oscilloscope. Lead 2 is likely to be the most useful for routine monitoring, though lead 3 will produce the most pronounced R-waves in cases of right axis deviation. Neonatal ECG moni-toring may be simplified by the use of a small back-plate with inbuilt electrodes.

It should be stressed that circulatory failure leading to hypoxic brain damage may occur before the ECG shows significant abnormalities.

Central venous pressure

Central venous pressure (CVP), which reflects right atrial filling pressure, expresses the relationship between the peripheral vascular resistance, blood volume and right heart function. Though CVP measurement must be interpreted with caution, it can provide a useful monitor of blood loss or blood replacement in the short term.

The internal jugular vein can be cannulated percutaneously in the neonate without great difficulty, using the technique described by English *et al.* (1964). The cannula is inserted through the junction of the medial one-third and lateral two-thirds of the sternomastoid muscle at a point mid-way between the mastoid process and the sternoclavicular joint, and directed towards the nipple. The vein, which is superficial in the infant, should be entered within 1–2 cm of the point of skin puncture, and can be made to fill and be more easily visualized by pressing over the liver. Care should be taken to avoid entering the common carotid artery, which lies just medial to the internal jugular vein at this point. If the cannula is inserted too far towards the thoracic inlet, puncture of the subclavian artery, the pleura or the lung may result. The subclavian vein has been safely cannulated by a percutaneous technique in the neonate. A skin incision is made below the clavicle, just lateral to its mid-point, and the needle is aimed at a point 1–1.5 cm above the sternal notch. The angle between the needle and the chest is initially about 45 degrees, enabling the needle to pass beneath the clavicle, when the angle is reduced to 15–20 degrees. If the infant has a prominent chest, the hub of the needle must be flattened against it during entry.

It is not possible to pass a central venous cannula percutaneously up the arm from the antecubital fossa in the neonate, though this can be done following surgical exposure.

The central venous cannula should be connected either to a simple water manometer or, via a short length of narrow-bore tubing, to a pressure transducer. It should be remembered that $1\,mmHg = 1.36\,cmH_2O$.

Left atrial pressure or pulmonary wedge pressure

Measurement of left atrial pressure is essential following repair of congenital heart lesions in the neonate because left atrial pressure gives a more reliable indication of blood loss or adequate replacement than right atrial or CVP pressure in this situation. Left atrial pressure lines can be inserted under direct vision at the time of operation by the surgeon, but care must be taken to ensure that air is not injected into them because this will be passed into the systemic circulation and may pass into the cerebral vessels. Following non-cardiac operations, pulmonary wedge pressure may be measured using the Swan–Ganz catheter inserted via the right internal jugular or subclavian vein. This measurement is sometimes used to monitor the effect of pulmonary vasodilating drugs in such conditions as congenital diaphragmatic hernia. It is, however, a difficult and potentially dangerous technique in the neonate and has little to offer over the continuous measurement of umbilical artery oxygen tension.

Fluid balance and blood replacement

The most accurate method of transfusion of blood or fluid in the newborn is by syringe, and the volume of fluid injected as diluent for muscle relaxants or other drugs should be included in the total fluid balance. The baby may arrive in the operating theatre with 100 ml measuring sets attached to the intravenous cannula, but these do not allow a rapid change from the administration of crystalloid fluids to blood.

Monitoring of blood loss is best achieved by weighing small numbers of swabs before they dry out. The experienced anaesthetist should also be able to make an approximate estimation of the blood loss from visual observation of the swabs. Allowance should be made for loss on drapes, and the volume of blood contained in the suction bottle should be measured directly. Colorimetric techniques are time consuming and do not allow the anaesthetist to obtain an estimate of blood loss at the time when it is occurring. Urine output may be monitored by the use of adhesive collecting bags, but in major surgery (such as cardiac surgery) catheterization should be performed.

Adequacy of volume replacement during surgery can be assessed by blood pressure, peripheral circulatory state or, in cases of massive blood replacement, by CVP monitoring. When blood is administered rapidly calcium should be given in a dose of 1 mmol·dl^{-1} blood.

Biochemical estimations

Biochemical estimations are seldom required during neonatal anaesthesia, though estimation of the blood glucose level is valuable in premature or small-for-dates infants. Dextrostix test strips are simple to use and reasonably reliable as long as they are fresh. In the sick hypoxic acidotic newborn, levels of serum calcium, sodium and potassium should be measured before surgery; blood gas and acid–base estimations may be needed, especially if cardiovascular failure ensues.

Temperature

Temperature should always be measured during neonatal surgery because of the increased susceptibility of the newborn to heat loss, and because hypothermia significantly increases morbidity and mortality. Nasopharyngeal, oesophageal or rectal temperatures can be most easily monitored and are all reliable though the latter temperature probe may become displaced during anaesthesia without the anaesthetist being aware of it.

Monitoring of theatre equipment

Anaesthetic machines

Anaesthetic machines and related equipment such as suction devices, upon which the patient's life may depend, must be thoroughly checked before anaesthesia is induced. This check includes inspection of the gas supply and breathing circuits, ensuring that pipeline probes are firmly inserted, that cylinders are full and are operating properly, a check of flowmeters and vaporizers, and a test to make sure there are no leaks in the circuit. Every anaesthetic machine should be equipped with an oxygen-failure alarm, and it is wise to have a simple oxygen analyser available in every operating theatre so that the oxygen concentration of inspired gas can be checked at any time.

Breathing circuits such as the T-piece should be fitted with pressure-release valves to ensure that pressures of more than 2–2.5 kPa (20–25 cmH$_2$O) cannot be applied to the airway. In addition, a heated humidifier should be available which can be incorporated into the circuit for long operations; the performance of the humidifier must be carefully monitored by measurement of the temperature of the inspired gas at the patient end of the circuit. Humidifiers must conform to accepted standards of electrical safety and a fail-safe cut-out device should operate in case of thermostat failure.

Mechanical ventilators

Mechanical ventilators should be fitted with an airway pressure gauge and expired volume meter such as a Wright's anemometer. Disconnection and overpressure alarms should also be provided in the circuit and these should have a built-in delay of 10–15 seconds to minimize disturbances caused by short periods of disconnection which are necessary for endotracheal suction or to empty water from the patient's circuit. In the operating theatre, most ventilators use a gas mixture provided from the flowmeters of the anaesthetic machine; when they are not, some form of monitor of inspired oxygen concentration should be incorporated in the circuit.

Heating devices

Because of the increased susceptibility of the newborn to heat loss, additional heat must be provided during anaesthesia and this is conventionally achieved by laying the baby on a heated electric or water blanket. These appliances must be electrically safe and must also be accurately monitored. Water mattresses must have an easily adjusted thermostat and a fail-safe cut-out device to prevent the water temperature rising above 42°C in the event of thermostat failure. The temperature difference between the heating unit and the water in the mattress depends on the length of connecting tubing and the circulating flow rate. It is therefore wise to monitor the temperature of the blanket by means of a thermistor probe placed between it and the skin surface of the neonate. Similar precautions should be taken with electrically heated blankets, and as an additional precaution it is wise for the anaesthetist to check the temperature of the blanket with his hand from time to time.

Environmental monitoring

Temperature

It is essential to monitor both the temperature and the rate of air change in the operating theatre during neonatal anaesthesia. The theatre should be draught-free and the temperature should be as high as can be tolerated by the staff. This latter is unlikely to be above 25°C.

Pollution

Increasing attention is being paid to the problems of pollution of the operating theatre by volatile and gaseous anaesthetic agents discharged from breathing circuits. The removal of these agents from the paediatric T-piece presents a particular problem. Though scavenging systems have been described which involve the insertion of collecting devices into the expiratory limb of the reservoir bag, or the modification of the circuit to include scavenged expiratory valves, these devices alter the basic simplicity of the T-piece, often make it more cumbersome to use and, in some cases, increase the danger of obstruction to expiratory gas flow. A scavenging dish (Fig. 3.17) for the anaesthetic T-piece which does not alter its characteristics has been described by Hatch, Miles and Wagstaff (1980). The dish removes large volumes of contaminated air and, if placed close to the open-tailed bag of the T-piece, provides a safe and convenient scavenger. It has been incorporated into a scavenging system which can also be used with a standard anti-pollution valve or ventilator exhaust port (Fig. 3.18). Measurements before and after installation have shown it to be capable of reducing nitrous oxide levels in the operating theatre to acceptable levels (Table 3.1). Levels of other anaesthetic gases or vapours such as halothane are known to follow nitrous oxide levels closely. Nitrous oxide is used in almost every anaesthetic given in the UK and levels are reasonably easy to measure because of the large volumes involved.

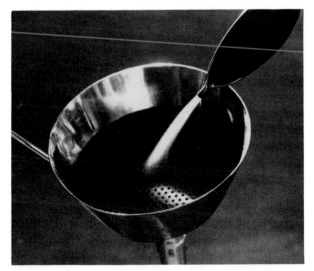

Fig. 3.17 A scavenging dish. Smoke is used to illustrate the effect of the scavenger on gas flow from the open tail of the T-piece bag. (From Hatch, Miles and Wagstaff, 1980)

Table 3.1 Maximum nitrous oxide levels obtained before and after scavenging

Operation	Age (yr)	Circuit	Ventilation	Maximum nitrous oxide levels (p.p.m.)		
				Anaesthetist's head	Patient's head	Surgeon's head
Before scavenging						
Femoral osteotomy	3½	T-piece	IPPV (manual)	620	850	120
Bat ears	8	Magill attachment	Spontaneous	185	320	300
Ureteric implantation	11½	Manley ventilator	IPPV	240	320	25
Urethroplasty	6/52	Sheffield ventilator	IPPV	700	1000+	240
After scavenging						
Cervical fusion	3	T-piece	IPPV (manual)	4–20	40	0
Hernia	1¼	T-piece	Spontaneous	0	0	0
Orchidopexy	8½	Magill attachment	Spontaneous	0	0	0

(From Hatch, Miles and Wagstaff, 1980)

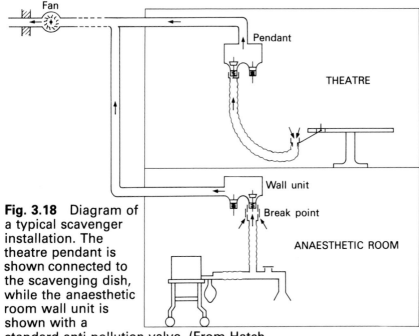

Fig. 3.18 Diagram of a typical scavenger installation. The theatre pendant is shown connected to the scavenging dish, while the anaesthetic room wall unit is shown with a standard anti-pollution valve. (From Hatch, Miles and Wagstaff, 1980)

References and further reading

Anaesthesia

Betts, E. K., Downes, J. J., Schaffer, D. B. and Johns, R. (1977). Retrolental fibroplasia and oxygen administration during general anesthesia. *Anesthesiology* **47**, 518.

Fisk, G. C. (1973). Equipment for inhalation anaesthesia for children. *Anaesthesia and Intensive Care* **1**, 468.

Goudsouzian, N. G. and Ryan, J. F. (1967). Recent advances in pediatric anesthesia. In: Symposium on Recent Clinical Advances. *Pediatric Clinics of North America* **23**, 345.

Gregory, G. A., Eger, E. I. and Munson, E. S. (1969). The relation between age and halothane requirements in man. *Anesthesiology* **30**, 488.

Hatch, D. J. (1978). Tracheal tubes and connectors used in neonates—dimensions and resistance to breathing. *British Journal of Anaesthesia* **50**, 959.

Katz, J. and Kadis, L. B. (Eds) (1973). *Anesthesia and Uncommon Diseases.* Saunders, Philadelphia and Eastbourne.

Kay, B. (1973). Neuroleptoanesthesia for neonates and infants. *Anesthesia and Analgesia* **52**, 970.

Koka, B. V., Jeon, I. S., Andre, J. M., Mackay, I. and Smith, R. M. (1977). Postintubation croup in children. *Anesthesia and Analgesia* **46**, 501.

Lomaz, J. G. (1965). Halothane and jaundice in paediatric anaesthesia. *Anaesthesia* **20**, 70.

Nightingale, D. A., Richards, C. C. and Glass, A. (1965). An evaluation of re-breathing in a modified T-piece system during controlled ventilation in anaesthetized children. *British Journal of Anaesthesia* **37**, 762.

Rashad, R. E. and Benson, D. W. (1967). Role of humidity in prevention of hypothermia in infants and children. *Anesthesia and Analgesia* **46**, 712.

Rayburn, R. L. and Graves, S. A. (1978). A new concept in controlled ventilation of children with the Bain anesthetic circuit. *Anesthesiology* **48**, 250.

Rees, G. J. (1958). Neonatal anaesthesia. *British Medical Bulletin* **14**, 38.

Rickham, P. P. (1954). An investigation of blood loss during operations on the newborn infant. *Archives of Disease in Childhood* **29**, 304.

Salanitre, E. and Rackow, H. (1969). The pulmonary exchange of nitrous oxide and halothane in infants and children. *Anesthesiology* 30, 388.

Salem, M. R., Wong, A. Y. and Collins, V. J. (1973). The pediatric patient with a full stomach. *Anesthesiology* **39**, 435.

Seeley, H. F., Barnes, P. K. and Conway, C. M. (1977). Controlled ventilation with the Mapleson D system. A theoretical and experimental study. *British Journal of Anaesthesia* **49**, 107.

Smith, P. C. and Smith, N. T. (1972). Anaesthetic management of a very premature infant. *British Journal of Anaesthesia* **44**, 736.

Steward, D. J. and Creighton, R. E. (1978). The uptake and excretion of nitrous oxide on the newborn. *Canadian Anaesthetists' Society Journal* **25**, 215.

Sumner, E. and Patrick, E. K. (1980). The Paediatric Patient, p. 359. In: *Preparation for Anaesthesia.* Ed. by A. J. Stevens, Pitman Medical, Tunbridge Wells.

Symposium on the Kidney and the Anaesthetist (1972). *British Journal of Anaesthesia* **44**, 236.

Symposium on Pediatric Anesthesia. (1975). *Anesthesiology* **43**, 141.

Symposium of Paediatric Anaesthesia and Intensive Care (1973). *Anaesthesia and Intensive Care* **1**, 457.

Vivori, E. and Bush, G. H. (1977). Modern aspects of the management of the newborn undergoing operation. *British Journal of Anaesthesia* **49**, 51.

Ward, R. J., Crawford, E. W. and Stevenson, J. K. (1970). Anesthetic experiences for infants under 2500 grams weight. *Anesthesia and Analgesia* **49**, 767.

Way, W. L., Costley, E. C. and Way, E. L. (1965). Respiratory sensitivity of the newborn infant to meperidine and morphine. *Clinical Pharmacology and Therapeutics* **6**, 454.

Willis, B. A., Pender, J. W. and Mapleson, W. W. (1975). Rebreathing in a T-piece: volunteer and theoretical studies of the Jackson Rees modification of the Ayre's T piece during spontaneous respiration. *British Journal of Anaesthesia* **47**, 1239.

Relaxants

Bennett, E. J., Ramanamurthy, S., Dalal, F. Y. and Salem, M. R. (1975). Pancuronium and the neonate. *British Journal of Anaesthesia* **47**, 75.

Bennett, E. J., Ignacio, A., Patel, K., Grundy, E. M. and Salem, M. R. (1976). Tubocurarine and the neonate. *British Journal of Anaesthesia* **48**, 687.

Bush G. H. and Stead A. L. (1962). The use of d-tubocurarine in neonatal anaesthesia. *British Journal of Anaesthesia* **34**, 721.

Churchill Davidson, H. C., Way, W. L. and de Jong, R. H. (1967). The muscle relaxants and renal excretion. *Anesthesiology* **28**, 540.

Goudsouzian, N. G., Donlon, J. V., Savarese, J. J. and Ryan, J. F. (1975). Re-evaluation of dosage and duration of action of *d*-tubocurarine in the pediatric age group. *Anesthesiology* **43**, 416.

Nightingale, D. A. and Bush, G. H. (1973). A clinical comparison between tubocurarine and pancuronium in children. *British Journal of Anaesthesia* **45**, 63.

Salem, M. R., Toyame, T., Wong, A. Y., Jacobs, H. K. and Bennett, E. J. (1977). Haemodynamic responses to antagonism of tubocurarine block with atropine prostigmine mixture in children. *British Journal of Anaesthesia* **49**, 901.

Watts, C. F. and Dillon, J. B. (1969). The response of newborn to succinyl choline and *d*-tubocurarine. *Anesthesiology* **31**, 35.

Zsigmond, E. K. and Downs, J. R. (1971). Plasma cholinesterase activity in newborns and infants. *Canadian Anaesthetists' Society Journal* **18**, 278.

Patient care during anaesthesia

Battersby, E. F. (1980). Monitoring during anesthesia for pediatric surgery. In: *International Anesthesiology Clinics*, Ed. by G. Gerson. Little, Brown & Co., Boston, Mass.

English, I. C. W., Frew, R. M., Piggott, J. F. and Zaki, M. (1964). Percutaneous catheterisation of the internal jugular vein. *Anaesthesia* **24**, 521.

Filston, H. C. and Grant, J. P. (1979). A safer system for percutaneous subclavian venous catheterization in newborn infants. *Journal of Pediatric Surgery* **14**, 564.

Furman, E. B., Hairabet, J. K. and Roman, D. G. (1972). The use of indwelling radial artery needles in paediatric anaesthesia. *British Journal of Anaesthesia* **44**, 531.

Hatch, D. J., Miles, R. and Wagstaff, M. (1980) An anaesthetic scavenging system for paediatric and adult use. *Anaesthesia* **35**, 496.

Saidman, L. J. and Smith, N. T. (1978). *Monitoring in Anesthesia*. Wiley, New York and Chichester.

4

Anaesthesia—
specific conditions

Surgical emergencies in the newborn

Almost all surgery in the neonatal period is performed on an emergency basis, and early diagnosis and treatment are essential if reasonable survival rates are to be achieved. The problems of transportation, preoperative assessment and general anaesthetic management of the neonate have already been discussed, and this chapter is devoted to specific surgical emergencies and their management.

Oesophageal atresia

Oesophageal atresia, with or without fistula, occurs in between 1 in 3000 and 1 in 3500 live births. In this condition, the main danger to life comes from the risk of aspiration of secretions into the bronchial tree, with subsequent pulmonary infection together with possible spill-over of acid gastric juice through the fistula. Although other factors will affect survival—particularly birth weight and the presence or absence of other major congenital abnormalities—early diagnosis and treatment before aspiration and contamination of the lungs has occurred is the factor where survival rates can be most improved by good management. The diagnosis should be suspected in any case of polyhydramnios and premature labour. At birth the baby is often seen to produce excess saliva which may drool from the mouth. The presence of oesophageal atresia can be confirmed by the inability to pass a soft no. 10 catheter down the oesophagus and into the stomach. If the catheter is too soft, it may coil in the upper pouch and the diagnosis may be missed. If a radio-opaque catheter is used, X-ray confirmation of the length of the blind ending upper pouch can be obtained. A plain X-ray of the chest and abdomen will also disclose the presence of a fistulous communication between the tracheobronchial tree and the lower oesophageal pouch, since any gas bubble seen in the stomach must have entered through such a communication (Fig. 4.1). Since the common anomaly is this combination of blind-ending upper pouch and lower pouch fistula (Fig. 4.2), the majority of cases of oesophageal atresia should be diagnosed easily soon after birth. The use of contrast medium is to be condemned because of the risk of pulmonary aspiration, compounding the pneumonitis and increasing the morbidity and mortality. The diagnosis of the rare upper pouch fistula is usually made by the surgeon at the time of operation, though some radiologists

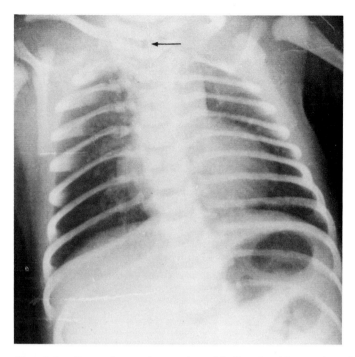

Fig. 4.1 Oesophageal atresia with fistula. X-ray showing opaque catheter in the upper pouch, aspiration pneumonitis and gas in the stomach.

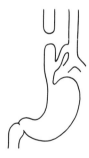

Fig. 4.2. Oesophageal atresia/fistula: the common anomaly (85 per cent incidence).

put a few drops of contrast medium into the upper pouch to exclude it (Fig. 4.3).

Perhaps the most difficult diagnosis to make is that of isolated tracheo-oesophageal fistula without oesophageal atresia. Prominent gaseous distension is often the presenting sign in the newborn but the diagnosis may be delayed for several months, when the infant usually presents with a history of recurrent attacks of chest infection. The differential diagnosis includes cystic fibrosis of the lungs, other causes of repeated aspiration such as inco-ordinated swallowing or hiatus hernia, and rare lung diseases. In this case diagnosis is usually made with the use of contrast media by a cine-oesophageal swallow. The films are sometimes difficult to interpret and they should be seen by an experienced radiologist.

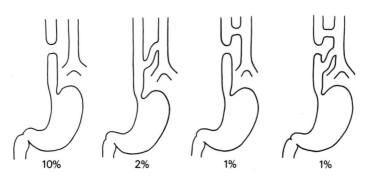

Fig. 4.3   Oesophageal atresia/fistula: the rarer anomalies (the approximate incidence is indicated under each).

Once the diagnosis of oesophageal atresia has been made, steps should be taken to protect the lungs from aspiration. The most satisfactory way of doing this is by the passage of a double-lumen Replogle tube into the upper pouch. Continuous low pressure suction is applied to one lumen and the second lumen entrains air, thus preventing the tube becoming stuck to the wall of the pouch. Alternatively, the upper pouch can be kept empty by intermittent suction. Gastro-oesophageal reflux is discouraged in the upright position but this position does not prevent the collection of mucus in the upper pouch and it may be preferable to nurse the baby prone. A delay of at least several hours with appropriate antibiotic therapy and physio-therapy may be justified before surgery, and has been shown to be of particular value where there has already been aspiration and contamination of the bronchial tree before the diagnosis has been made.

Associated anomalies

More than half the babies presenting with oesophageal atresia have associ-ated congenital anomalies. The most common are congenital heart disease, other upper airway problems, renal, genitourinary and additional gastro-intestinal anomalies such as anorectal agenesis. Vertebral and skeletal abnormalities also frequently occur. These babies are commonly of low birth weight, and Waterston in 1962 showed that mortality rose steeply with low birth weight, the presence of other major anomalies and severity of pneumonia (Waterson, Bonham Carter and Aberdeen, 1962). They de-scribed three groups of patients with differing survival rates classified according to these factors. Group A, with lowest mortality (5 per cent), comprised babies of birth weight over 2.5 kg who were well. Group B, with a mortality of 32 per cent, comprised babies weighing 1.8–2.5 kg and those of higher birth weight with moderate pneumonia or congenital anomalies. Group C, with the highest mortality at 94 per cent, comprised babies weighing under 1.8 kg and those of higher birth weight with severe pneumonia or congenital anomalies.

Anaesthetic management

It is not necessary for endotracheal intubation to be performed before arrival in the operating theatre; this is usually carried out awake as for any other neonatal surgical emergency, though the upper pouch should be aspirated and the double-lumen Replogle tube removed immediately before intubation. When the endotracheal tube has been secured in place, the lungs should be gently inflated and careful auscultation of the chest carried out to ensure that adequate air entry is achieved in both lungs. The stethoscope should also be placed over the stomach to check that the anaesthetic gases are not inflating it via the fistula. In the majority of cases the lungs can be adequately inflated without distension of the stomach, but if the position of the endotracheal tube is not satisfactory, it is usually because the tip is pointing towards the fistula. It is extremely unusual to intubate the fistula itself, though this has been reported. If a significant amount of gas is passing through the fistula, the endotracheal tube should be repositioned, either by withdrawing it slightly, passing it further down the trachea, or by turning it on its connector so that its bevelled tip is pointing in a different direction. It is unusual not to be able to find a position where the lungs can be satisfactorily inflated without a significant amount of air passing through the fistula, and normally controlled ventilation can be commenced with the use of muscle relaxants. In the unlikely event of it not being possible to inflate the lungs adequately, or if the stomach is being significantly distended, the surgeon should be informed and the patient allowed to continue to breathe spontaneously. Most surgeons would perform gastrostomy before thoracotomy in this rare situation, and some surgeons prefer to do this for every case, as it prevents the risk of the enlarging stomach splinting the diaphragm and impeding respiration further. When the chest is opened, controlled ventilation must be commenced, and if adequate inflation of the lungs is not achieved, the surgeon should control the leak through the fistula as soon as possible—if necessary, using his finger to do this in the first instance. The normal approach to the fistula is extrapleural, though this takes longer and cannot be used in the emergency described above.

The other problem which the anaesthetist is likely to face is surgical retraction during the thoracotomy, which may obstruct ventilation. If the lungs are already stiff with severe pneumonia, it may be difficult to detect complete obstruction, but in most cases the sudden change in pressure required to inflate the lungs is easily detected by the hand. For this reason, manual ventilation is preferred to mechanical ventilation. The use of the precordial stethoscope is extremely valuable in these cases, particularly for the information it provides about the amount of air entering the lungs.

Occasionally the trachea can be seriously damaged during the surgery and large air leaks may occur.

Anaesthesia can be maintained with 50 per cent nitrous oxide/50 per cent oxygen, with the addition of halothane if required. Non-depolarizing or depolarizing muscle relaxants can be used. Blood should be available for transfusion, but with experienced surgical care it is seldom required. Usually, sufficient crystalloid solution is given with the various diluted drugs administered to satisfy maintenance requirements, which are low in the first few days of life (as described on p. 32).

The upper pouch should be sucked from time to time and occasionally tracheobronchial suction may be required.

Postoperative care

Postoperatively, if the chest is not seriously contaminated and the patient is awake and moving vigorously with no residual effects of muscle relaxation, extubation can be performed. If there is any doubt about the adequacy of ventilation, however, or if the lungs are seriously contaminated, it is probably wiser to continue controlled ventilation for at least 24 hours. These babies all need intensive postoperative care; even in conservative centres, approximately 25 per cent of them will need some period of postoperative ventilation. Intragastric feeding is commenced as soon as possible, either via a transanastomotic feeding tube or by gastrostomy.

If, for anatomical reasons, primary anastomosis of the two ends of the oesophagus cannot be achieved, a feeding gastrostomy will be performed and continuous suction must be applied to the upper pouch until a delayed repair can be performed.

Anaesthesia for oesophagoscopy

After primary anastomosis of oesophageal atresia, repeated oesophageal dilatations may be necessary for actual or incipient strictures.

Premedication is with atropine, and awake intubation with a 3 mm Oxford tube or 2.5 mm plain red rubber tube with curved Magill connection is performed after preoxygenation. If anaesthesia is required in an older baby, the use of cricoid pressure must be considered to prevent aspiration of regurgitated upper oesophageal contents. The T-piece comes down over the baby's chest. A relaxant technique with controlled ventilation is most satisfactory and intermittent suxamethonium is possibly the relaxant of choice. The eyes must be protected by taping, and heart beat and respiration monitored with a precordial stethoscope. The passage of the oesophagoscope may compress the trachea and obstruct the ventilation. Coughing on the endotracheal tube when the oesophagoscope is in place has been responsible for oesophageal perforations, so perfect immobility should be produced throughout. After the endoscopy the patient is allowed to awaken fully, suction is carefully applied to the pharynx and extubation performed with the infant on his side.

Congenital diaphragmatic hernia

Congenital diaphragmatic hernia is a rare but serious emergency in the newborn period, with an incidence of approximately 1 in 4000 live births. There are several types of anomaly, the commonest occurring through a posterolateral defect in the left side of the diaphragm at the foramen of Bochdalek. The hernia usually consists of the whole of the mid-gut, and may include the stomach, part of the descending colon, the left kidney, the spleen and the left lobe of the liver. The mid-gut fills with air soon after birth—usually at the time of the first feed—causing displacement of the mediastinum to the right and compression of the right lung (Fig. 4.4).

The onset of respiratory distress depends largely on the degree of pulmonary hypoplasia present, which may be ipsilateral or bilateral. Those babies who develop respiratory distress within the first 4 hours of life have a very high mortality, and lung weights on the affected side may be found at

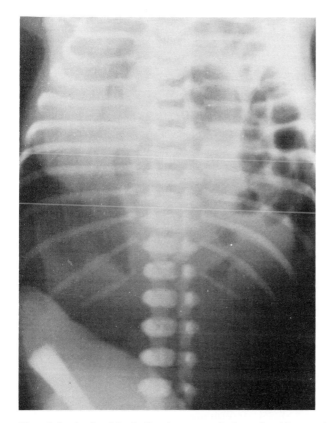

Fig. 4.4 Left-sided diaphragmatic hernia. X-ray showing gross mediastinal displacement caused by gas-filled intestine in the left chest.

post-mortem to be as low as 2 g compared with a normal individual lung weight of from 17 to 35 g in full-term babies. Combined lung weights are often low, even when compared with babies of similar gestational age. In some babies, congenital diaphragmatic hernia causes little respiratory embarrassment, and occasionally the diagnosis is not made until early childhood or even later. These children presumably have little or no pulmonary hypoplasia. The reason why some cases of diaphragmatic hernia have severe pulmonary hypoplasia and others apparently very little is not clear. Work in animals suggests that it depends upon the gestational age at which herniation of the intestinal contents into the chest actually occurs (Fig. 4.5). If lung maturation is arrested by the herniation, it is clear that when this occurs early in intrauterine life there is a greater chance of pulmonary hypoplasia than when it occurs later.

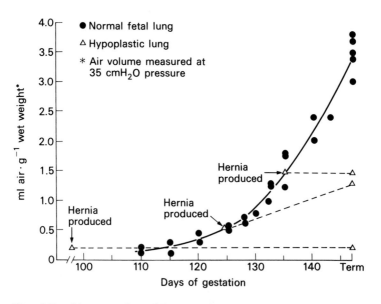

Fig. 4.5   Air capacity of lungs of lambs at gestational ages 110–147 days. The lungs of lambs with diaphragmatic hernia had air capacities equivalent to lungs at the gestational age at which the hernia was produced. (From de Lorimer *et al.,* 1967)

Associated anomalies

The problem of associated pulmonary hypoplasia is discussed above. Other lung anomalies such as sequestrated pulmonary lobes also occur.

The commonest anomalies associated with diaphragmatic hernia are intestinal ones, particularly malrotation of the gut. Congenital heart disease and renal anomalies are less common.

Diagnosis

Congenital diaphragmatic hernia should be suspected in any case of respiratory distress occurring soon after birth. Examination of the chest may reveal reduced movement and reduced breath sounds on the affected side, dullness to percussion, mediastinal displacement and a scaphoid abdomen. A straight X-ray will usually confirm the diagnosis although this can occasionally be confused with congenital pulmonary lobar emphysema.

Anaesthetic management

The onset of respiratory distress with severe hypoxia soon after birth demands urgent treatment, usually by endotracheal intubation and ventilation, though deflation of the stomach through a nasogastric tube usually helps. The lungs should not be inflated with a face mask since this will increase the amount of air passing into the stomach and intestines and thus increase the mediastinal displacement. Urgent laparotomy to reduce the hernia is essential to survival in these severely ill babies, and the intubated ventilated child should be transferred to the operating theatre as soon as possible. An intravenous line should be inserted, and if possible an arterial sample should be obtained so that any metabolic acidosis can be corrected. This should not, however, delay surgery because the child's condition is unlikely to improve until the hernia has been reduced. For the same reason, the operation should not be delayed while blood is cross-matched. In view of the possibility of pulmonary hypoplasia, great care should be taken not to use excessive pressures when ventilating the lungs, as these may cause alveolar rupture and pneumothorax. If possible, inflating pressure should be kept below 25–30 cmH$_2$O. The possibility of a pneumothorax on the contralateral side should always be borne in mind and drainage of the pleural cavity should always be considered if the baby's condition suddenly deteriorates. No attempt should be made to expand the ipsilateral lung at the end of the operation, as this manoeuvre will almost certainly cause a pneumothorax.

ECG, blood pressure and nasopharyngeal temperature should be monitored continuously throughout the operation. The use of a precordial stethoscope may be impracticable if it interferes with the surgical field. If the baby has required preoperative ventilation, or if the operation has been performed within 24 hours of birth, postoperative ventilatory support is almost certain to be needed; in these cases it is wise to continue ventilation for at least 24 hours postoperatively and to insert an umbilical or radial artery catheter for blood gas measurements at the end of the operation. Older babies who have not required preoperative respiratory support and who are breathing satisfactorily at the end of surgery may be extubated, but it is wise to return all babies to the ward breathing an oxygen-enriched mixture.

Postoperative care

As stated above, babies presenting with respiratory distress within the first few hours of birth are likely to need preoperative, intraoperative and postoperative ventilatory support, and many of these will remain hypoxic postoperatively owing to pulmonary hypoplasia despite controlled ventilation with high oxygen mixtures. If the immaturity of the lungs is so great as to be incompatible with life, no amount of intensive postoperative care will save the child. There are, however, a group of babies who can be saved by these techniques despite severe immaturity of the lungs. Some of these babies tend to revert to a fetal circulation with right-to-left shunting through the patent ductus arteriosus, and in these the use of pulmonary vasodilators such as tolazoline hydrochloride may be considered. This can either be infused into the pulmonary artery or given systemically in a dose of 1 mg·kg^{-1} body weight. Attempts should be made to keep arterial oxygen tension between 8 and 10.7 kPa (60–80 mmHg) free gastric drainage and intravenous administration of fluids should be continued until normal bowel action commences, and the possibility of sudden pneumothorax should be anticipated.

Exomphalos and gastroschisis

Exomphalos is a herniation into the umbilical cord and gastroschisis is a defect of the abdominal wall lateral to the umbilicus, usually on the right side. The exomphalos sac may be intact or may rupture before, during or after birth with prolapsed abdominal contents coming through it; on the other hand, the gastroschisis is always ruptured *in utero* and has no covering membrane. Exomphalos, with an incidence of between 1 in 5000 and 1 in 10 000 live births, is more common than gastroschisis, which has an approximate incidence of 1 in 30 000 live births. There is evidence that gastroschisis is becoming more common.

Associated anomalies

The common associated anomalies are other gastrointestinal or craniofacial anomalies, including hare lip and cleft palate, genitourinary anomalies and congenital heart disease. Many of these babies are of low birth weight, particularly those with gastroschisis. Exomphalos forms parts of the Beckwith–Wiedemann syndrome (p. 188).

Anaesthetic management.   Surgical treatment is usually by excision of the sac when present and repair of the anterior abdominal wall. Most anaesthetic problems arise from impaired ventilation if closure of the abdominal wall compresses the intestinal contents, pushing the diaphragm upwards and restricting its downward movement on inspiration. This may occur even with full muscle relaxation. The recent use of a pouch of Silastic to augment the abdominal wall temporarily in the severest cases has alleviated the problem for the anaesthetist, as the intestinal contents are gradually returned to the abdominal cavity during the course of the first few days of life. There is a risk, however, that the edges of the Silastic pouch may tear away from the abdominal wall, or may become infected, and the use of Silastic can now often be avoided by manual stretching of the abdominal skin.

Other anaesthetic problems arise from severe fluid and electrolyte disturbances resulting from transudation of bowel fluid and from heat loss from
the large exposed visceral surfaces.

Postoperative care

Relatively few cases of exomphalos need postoperative respiratory support,
and mortality in this condition is largely due to associated major congenital
anomalies.

In gastroschisis, ventilation and mortality rates remain fairly high despite
advances in surgical treatment such as the use of the Silastic pouch described
above. The bowel wall has usually become thickened because of its exposure
to amniotic fluid, and the onset of peristalsis is often delayed. Continuous
intravenous feeding is often required for up to 6 weeks or so in this condition
and this has significantly improved survival rates, though there is a risk that
central feeding lines may become infected, leading to septicaemia, particularly from organisms such as *Candida*. Continuous nasogastric suction
should be performed during this period, and electrolyte and acid–base status
regularly checked.

Intestinal obstruction

Intestinal obstruction is one of the commonest surgical emergencies in the
newborn, amounting to approximately 25 per cent of all neonatal emergency operations. Though the chemical composition of the neonate with
congenital intestinal obstruction is normal at birth, delay in diagnosis will
cause increasing fluid and electrolyte disturbances. In addition, increasing
abdominal distension may lead to respiratory embarrassment and the risk of
aspiration. Aspiration pneumonitis has been a common early cause of
death, which may occur before other complications have time to arise. The
passage of a gastric tube before transfer to a neonatal surgical unit is
mandatory. Dehydration, shock and acidosis may complicate the picture,
together with the possibility of intestinal perforation and septicaemia due to
ischaemic necrosis of obstructed bowel. Finally, the high incidence of associated major congenital anomalies also increases the mortality and morbidity.
The fact that a low overall mortality can be achieved in this group of patients
(Table 4.1) is largely related to early diagnosis and treatment.

The possibility of intestinal obstruction should be borne in mind in cases
of toxaemia of pregnancy, polyhydramnios and premature labour, and
where there is a family history of such diseases as mucoviscidosis or Hirschsprung's disease. The likelihood of obstruction—organic or functional—
becomes very high when there is green-stained vomiting by the baby, or
failure to pass meconium for 24 hours.

Duodenal atresia

Duodenal obstruction may be due to complete atresia, stenosis, intraluminal diaphragm or annular pancreas. The reported incidence is between 1 in

Table 4.1   Admissions to a neonatal surgical unit 1974–1977

Diagnosis	No.	Deaths	
Abdominal surgery:			
General	165	14	(8.5%)
Exomphalos	22	2	(9.1%)
Gastroschisis	15	5	(33.3%)
Tracheo-oesophageal fistula/atresia	69	9	(13.0%)
Diaphragmatic hernia	36	13	(36.1%)
Miscellaneous	18	4	(22.2%)
Total	325	47	(14.5%)
Meningomyelocele	53	2	(3.8%)

6000 and 1 in 20 000 live births. The stomach and proximal duodenum dilate rapidly, giving rise to the classic 'double bubble' on erect X-ray (Fig. 4.6). Vomiting usually occurs early, and becomes copious and forceful. If the obstruction is below the ampulla of Vater, vomiting will become bile-stained, but many cases of duodenal atresia are supra-ampullary. Later, hypochloraemic alkalosis, weight loss and dehydration may occur. Gastric perforation has been reported.

Associated anomalies.   About 70 per cent of cases have one or more associated congenital anomalies. One-third have Down's syndrome (mongolism), often itself associated with congenital heart disease; 15 per cent have cystic fibrosis. Other intestinal anomalies, such as malrotation, oesophageal atresia, imperforate anus and Meckel's diverticulum, are fairly common, as are renal anomalies. Fifty per cent of these neonates weigh less than 2.5 kg at birth, and 20 per cent less than 2 kg.

Anaesthetic problems.   Since these neonates are generally operated upon within 3 days of birth, their general condition is usually quite good. They may, however, have evidence of pneumonitis or atelectasis from pulmonary aspiration. Gastric distension may be splinting the diaphragm and should be relieved with a nasogastric tube. The surgical procedure, usually duodeno-duodenostomy, requires full muscle relaxation but otherwise presents few problems to the anaesthetist. Blood loss is usually slight, and transfusion seldom required.

Late cases may present with dehydration, hypothermia, shock and severe metabolic and electrolyte disturbances.

Other atresias

With an incidence of between 1 in 1500 and 1 in 3000 live births, other atresias are usually jejunal or ileal, and occasionally colonic. Multiple atresias occur in about 10 per cent of cases. In some the intestine is arranged

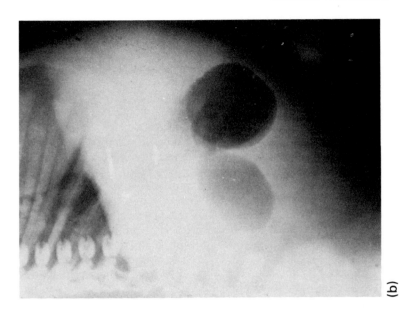

(b)

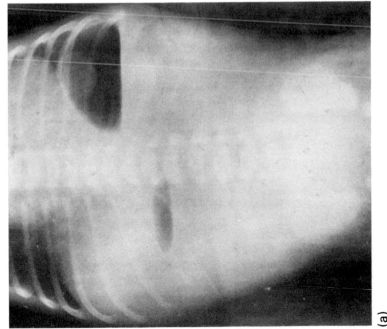

(a)

Fig. 4.6 Duodenal atresia. (a) Posteroanterior and (b) lateral erect X-rays showing the classic 'double bubble'.

in a spiral around a central mesenteric vessel, and is known as 'apple peel' or 'maypole' atresia. These cases tend to have a familial incidence.

Whatever the cause, the proximal intestine dilates enormously and this may interfere with venous return from the bowel, causing bowel wall congestion or necrosis. Bile-stained vomiting occurs earlier with high lesions. Meconium peritonitis is present in approximately 30 per cent of cases, probably secondary to bowel infarction.

Associated anomalies. These are mainly other intestinal abnormalities such as volvulus. Birth weights are often within the normal range.

Anaesthetic problems. The main anaesthetic problems are respiratory embarrassment or aspiration from the gross distension that sometimes occurs, particularly with atresias low in the intestinal tract. The volume and complexity of the composition of fluid lost are also greater with low atresias. Intestinal losses should be replaced with normal saline, though bicarbonate may also be needed to correct any metabolic acidosis. Increased capillary permeability causes loss of crystalloid and colloid from vessels in the bowel wall; if shock is present, colloid up to $20 \, \text{ml} \cdot \text{kg}^{-1}$ should be infused rapidly. This is more likely to occur with low obstructions, where the diagnosis may have been delayed and bowel infarction, meconium peritonitis or bacterial peritonitis may be present. Gaseous distension may be made worse by the use of nitrous oxide, and severe metabolic derangement may potentiate the action of the muscle relaxants.

Malrotations and volvulus

Considering how complicated the process of rotation of the intestine is in the normal fetus, it is perhaps not surprising that things may go wrong and the gut may take up a number of abnormal positions. The commonest one is for the duodenum to lie behind or to the right of the superior mesenteric artery with the caecum in front of it. Folds of peritoneum, known as Ladd's bands, attach the caecum to the posterior abdominal wall, in the right hypochondrium, and these tend to obstruct the second part of the duodenum (Fig. 4.7). Malrotations are, however, surprisingly rare.

If intestinal strangulation occurs due to volvulus, blood may be passed per rectum, and abdominal distension will ensue as with other causes of intestinal obstruction.

Associated anomalies. Exomphalos and duodenal atresia are sometimes associated with malrotation as is diaphragmatic hernia.

Anaesthetic problems. The problems are either those of partial duodenal obstruction or of volvulus, where distension and fluid and electrolyte losses secondary to vomiting occur early. The situation may be complicated by pyrexia, bowel infarction or septicaemia. Surgery usually only involves division of Ladd's bands, derotation and fixation of the bowel, but occasionally resection of non-viable bowel and creation of a double-barrelled

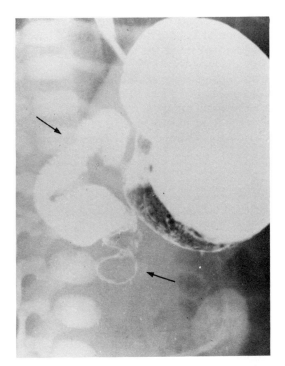

Fig. 4.7   Volvulus. Barium X-ray showing obstruction to the second part of the duodenum by Ladd's bands and the classic twisted ribbon sign.

enterostomy is required. In the worse cases the amount of viable bowel left may be incompatible with life.

It has been claimed that the incidence of bowel necrosis can be reduced by the use of low molecular weight dextran. Similar claims have been made in animals for the use of hyperbaric oxygen, but these have not been substantiated in man.

Meconium ileus

Between 10 and 15 per cent of patients with cystic fibrosis (mucoviscidosis) present with meconium ileus, which has an incidence of about 1 in 20 000 live births. In this condition, the distal ileum is obstructed by inspissated meconium with a consistency similar to chewing gum. Atresias, volvulus, perforation, gangrene and meconium peritonitis are common complications.

A Gastrografin enema, containing the wetting agent Tween 80, may relieve obstruction in selected uncomplicated cases, but since complications are sometimes hard to detect many people prefer surgery in all cases. At laparotomy, the distal ileum is often found to be distended, and surgery may involve resection of non-viable segments of bowel and the creation of ileostomy. In addition, Tween 80 injected into the bowel lumen may enable some of the sticky meconium to be milked out of the cut end of the bowel, but too much handling of the bowel may make the situation worse.

Anaesthetic problems.   These are related to the degree of obstruction and the presence of the complications mentioned above. The use of atropine is controversial, as it may increase the viscid nature of tracheal secretions. In addition, the respiratory problems of cystic fibrosis mean that careful attention must be given to humidifying the respired gases, especially in the postoperative period.

Milk plug obstruction

This rare cause of lower ileal obstruction is due to a mass of inspissated milk, and is seen only in babies reared on artificial feeds. The baby is normal at birth, passes normal meconium and stools, and then develops intestinal obstruction, possibly due to transient reduction in bile acid excretion.

Surgery is usually required, but seldom involves more than milking the obstruction through the ileocaecal valve into the caecum.

Meconium plugs

Meconium plugs are often associated with Hirschsprung's disease, and are usually removed by rectal washouts.

Duplication cysts

These are rare, but can occur anywhere from the tongue to the anus. Intrathoracic duplications may cause respiratory distress and mediastinal shift as they fill with secretions. Perforation or ulceration into the oesophagus or bronchus has been reported, but this seldom occurs in the neonatal period.

Abdominal duplications may mimic pyloric stenosis, become the starting points of an intussusception, cause intestinal obstruction by ribboning or by volvulus, perforate or bleed.

Hirschsprung's disease

This disease involves a functional obstruction due to lack of ganglia in the distal colon and rectum. The incidence is probably between 1 in 5000 and 1 in 10 000 live births, though varying figures have been reported.

In most cases vomiting, reluctance to feed and abdominal distension begin within 48 hours of birth. There is commonly failure to pass meconium, and erect X-ray shows multiple fluid levels typical of low intestinal obstruction (Fig. 4.8). Barium enema or anorectal manometry studies may help in establishing the diagnosis, but rectal suction biopsy is required for confirmation.

Rectal washouts may temporarily relieve the obstruction, but colostomy

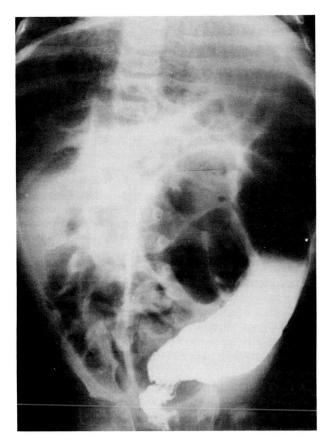

Fig. 4.8 Hirschsprung's disease. X-ray using radio-opaque medium to demonstrate the zone of transition at the sigmorectal level.

is usually performed in the neonatal period, followed by a 'pull-through' operation 6–9 months later to bring the ganglionated bowel through the preserved sphincteric mechanisms to the perineum.

Anaesthetic problems. In the neonate there are usually few anaesthetic problems, though occasionally older children may present for surgery with gross abdominal distension and general debility. Neonatal problems are related to recurrent intestinal obstruction and the development of potentially fatal complications such as necrotizing enterocolitis.

Intussusception

Intussusception rarely occurs in the neonate, except in the presence of duplication cysts. Intrauterine intussusception has been reported as a cause of intestinal atresias.

Anorectal anomalies

These result from an embryological failure of differentiation of the cloaca and urogenital sinus. They are divided into 'high' anomalies (rectal agenesis), when the rectum ends above the levator muscle, and 'low' anomalies (covered anus), when it passes through the muscle to end close to the perineum. High anomalies, often accompanied by a rectourethral fistula are commoner than low anomalies in the male. In the female, high anomalies, often accompanied by a rectovaginal fistula, are rarer than low ones.

Associated anomalies.   Over 60 per cent of babies with anorectal anomalies, particularly high ones, have one or more associated anomalies. Genitourinary anomalies are most common, because of the closely integrated embryology of the two systems. Vertebral and skeletal anomalies and congenital heart defects are also common, as are alimentary tract anomalies, particularly oesophageal atresia and Hirschsprung's disease.

Anaesthetic problems.   Most of the anaesthetic problems are related to the associated anomalies. The surgical management of the covered anus is by the relatively simple procedure of anal 'cut-back' performed in the lithotomy position, whilst high rectal agenesis is usually treated by colostomy at birth followed by a definitive 'pull-through' procedure 6–9 months later.

Caudal analgesia has been recommended for these procedures, using 0.25 per cent bupivacaine without adrenaline (1 ml·kg^{-1}). Onset of analgesia takes 15–20 minutes, but is more rapid if 1 per cent lignocaine is added to the bupivacaine.

Congenital pyloric stenosis

This is one of the commonest malformations of the digestive tract, its incidence having been estimated at between 1 in 300 and 1 in 400 live births. Approximately 85 per cent of affected infants are male, and between 40 and 60 per cent are first borns. The pathological abnormality is a gross thickening of the circular muscle of the pylorus, which forms a hard tumour and causes an increasing degree of obstruction to the passage of food from the stomach. The presenting symptom is vomiting, which does not usually start before the tenth day, but increases in severity and generally becomes projectile. The infant loses weight and becomes dehydrated, and loss of chloride from the stomach may produce hypochloraemic alkalosis and even tetany. The physical signs which confirm the presence of pyloric stenosis are visible gastric peristalsis, especially after feeds (though this is an unreliable physical sign) and the presence of a palpable tumour usually felt just to the right of the umbilicus. The absence of a palpable tumour does not, however, exclude the diagnosis and radiological examination can also be misleading. Whilst medical treatment has been advocated in this condition, it is now general practice to recommend surgical correction by pyloromyotomy in virtually every case. This operation is not, however, an emergency procedure and must be preceded by complete correction of fluid and electrolyte abnormalities. There is a total loss of sodium chloride (chloride lost by vomiting and sodium in combination with bicarbonate by the kidneys). Potassium is also lost by a renal attempt to conserve sodium and hydrogen ion. The extent of the K^+ loss is not usually well reflected in serum levels. A compensatory respiratory acidosis is also seen, with hypoventilation to the point of apnoea. Extremes of dehydration are rare nowadays, but would be seen with prolonged vomiting when pH falls with keto-acidosis and when a vicious circle develops with falling cardiac output, increasing acidosis and hypoxia.

No surgery should be undertaken until the chloride is at least 90 mmol·l^{-1} and the bicarbonate 24 mmol·l^{-1}; 0.9 per cent sodium chloride may be given and up to 400 ml may be necessary. (Giving 0.9 per cent NaCl 2 ml·kg^{-1} will raise the chloride by 1 mmol·l^{-1}.) Most cases are diagnosed early nowadays, however, and little fluid or electrolyte replacement therapy is required.

Maintenance fluids should be 2 ml·kg^{-1} per hour of 4 per cent dextrose in 0.18 per cent saline. Mild cases do not need potassium supplements, but in others it should be given at a rate not exceeding 3 mmol·kg^{-1} per 24 hours. A large gastric residue is drained off and 4-hourly washouts of the stomach with normal saline are carried out until the aspirate is clear and odourless (a secondary gastritis is often present).

Atropine premedication is given and the nasogastric tube aspirated before induction of anaesthesia. The tube will be left in place because it does not reduce the effectiveness of cricoid pressure and will act as a 'blow off' valve if the intragastric pressure should rise.

The patients are usually too old and too lusty for awake intubation so consideration must be paid to a possible risk of regurgitation of stomach contents and their subsequent aspiration during the induction of anaesthesia. This is extremely unlikely if the nasogastric tube is left open after aspiration.

Induction of anaesthesia is by an inhalation or by an intravenous method. Cricoid pressure is as effective in babies as it is in adults and may be applied after suxamethonium has been given for relaxation. Intermittent suxamethonium (increments of 5 mg) has been described as the relaxant of choice for the operation of pyloromyotomy, but equally good conditions can be obtained using small doses of tubocurarine.

The surgical procedure involves delivering the pylorus, splitting the muscle and then closing the abdomen. It is important that the child does not cough or strain at the time of muscle splitting, as the surgeon is attempting to cut down to but not through the mucosa. Postoperative morbidity increases if the mucosal layer is incised. The baby should be extubated awake in the lateral position.

Postoperative care

Oral feeding with clear fluids can usually be started 4–6 hours after the operation, but an intravenous infusion of 4 per cent dextrose in 0.18 per cent saline (3 ml·kg^{-1} per hour) should be maintained for the first 12–24 hours until a normal oral intake has been re-established.

Biliary atresia

Biliary atresia may be extrahepatic, or, more commonly, intrahepatic, and other major congenital anomalies such as congenital heart disease may be associated. Surgical exploration of the bile ducts and intraoperative cholangiography are usually required to confirm the exact nature of the anomaly and to assess the feasibility of surgical correction by some form of anastomosis between the porta hepatis or biliary passages and the intestinal tract.

Anaesthetic management

These babies may have coagulation abnormalities, and haematological studies should be carried out before surgery. It is probably wise to administer 1 mg vitamin K_1 intramuscularly prior to surgery, as hypoprothrombinaemia is common. The other major problem which may be encountered is blood loss; this can be substantial, so a reliable intravenous line must be inserted and adequate supplies of blood must be available for transfusion if required.

Inguinal hernia

Inguinal hernias may present towards the end of the neonatal period; because these may become incarcerated, repair should not be delayed. The hernia is usually the result of a patent processus vaginalis and repair is by simple herniotomy. Most hernias can be reduced easily at this age and it is unusual for the patient to develop significant intestinal obstruction provided diagnosis and treatment are carried out without delay.

Anaesthetic management

If strangulation has occurred, the baby may be shocked and dehydrated with loss of water and electrolytes by vomiting. Such babies must be treated by nasogastric suction and intravenous therapy before surgery. The main problem arising at operation is that traction on the peritoneum is extremely stimulating to the child and may cause laryngeal spasm if endotracheal intubation has not been performed. For this reason intubation is recommended, but the procedure can be conducted using spontaneous or controlled ventilation. The child should be allowed to wake up before extubation is performed.

Postoperative care

If the child's general condition is satisfactory, a graduated feeding regimen can be started after a few hours, as for pyloric stenosis.

Postoperative analgesia is seldom required at this age but intramuscular codeine phosphate in a dose of $1 \, mg \cdot kg^{-1}$ can be safely used.

Cystic hygroma

This cystic lymphangioma presents at birth as a multiloculated cystic swelling in the neck (Fig. 4.9) or, rarely, in the axilla. The swelling is soft and fluctuant, and although it is benign it frequently invades neighbouring tissues and may recur. It may not be possible to perform complete surgical removal, especially if the tumour is large or extends around the trachea or brachial plexus. Involvement of the base of the tongue and oropharynx is common and may cause respiratory difficulties. Intrathoracic extension of this tumour is rare.

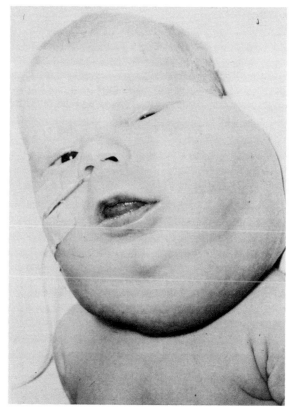

Fig. 4.9 Cystic hygroma.

Anaesthetic management

The intraoral extension of this multilocular cystic tumour may make identification of the larynx difficult and, more importantly, may make inflation of the lungs impossible in the apnoeic patient. It is therefore essential to maintain spontaneous breathing until intubation has been performed. In the worst cases the only way to identify the larynx may be to observe the movement of air in and out of the lungs, which usually causes a small number of frothy bubbles to appear between two lobules of the hygroma. The surgical removal of the tumour may be difficult and blood should be available for transfusion. The child should not be extubated until fully awake, and in the worst cases tracheostomy may be required.

Postoperative care

Because of the danger of bleeding into the operative site causing respiratory obstruction in the early postoperative period, these children must be observed closely. Even the aperture of a tracheostomy tube may become obstructed by recurrent swelling in the neck.

Congenital lobar emphysema

Although rare, this condition may present as a cause of serious respiratory distress in the newborn period. The emphysematous lobe, which is commonly the left upper, right upper or right middle lobe, compresses the normal lung tissue and may displace the mediastinum (Fig. 4.10).

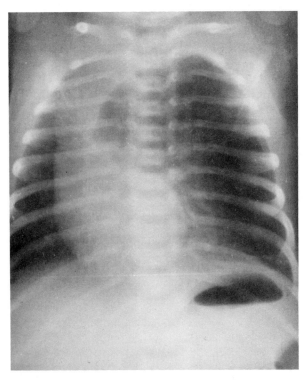

Fig. 4.10 Congential lobar emphysema. X-ray showing mediastinal displacement to the right.

Associated anomalies

The condition is frequently associated with congenital heart disease.

Anaesthetic management

These children may present either for bronchoscopy or lobectomy, though bronchoscopy is not usually indicated and is dangerous in the presence of intrapleural tension problems. The only safe way of performing bronchoscopy is with spontaneous ventilation, and the bronchoscope should be passed under fairly deep anaesthesia, usually with halothane. The laryngeal inlet and upper trachea can be sprayed with lignocaine with a maximum dose of 4 mg·kg^{-1}. If the surgeon decides to proceed to lobectomy, the bronchoscope should be removed and an endotracheal tube inserted. Care should be taken with controlled ventilation because of the risk of making the emphysematous lobe even more distended, or producing pneumothorax. However, once the chest is opened it is essential that controlled ventilation is applied and this is best performed with full muscle relaxation. Cullum, English and Branthwaite (1973) have described a technique for endobronchial intubation in this condition. It may be necessary to leave an endotracheal tube in place postoperatively, but if it is to be removed, this should not be done until the patient is fully awake.

Postoperative care

The infant should be nursed in an oxygen-enriched environment in a head box, and a postoperative chest X-ray should be taken to confirm adequate expansion of the remaining areas of lung.

Since this condition is sometimes associated with generalized chondromalacia of the bronchial walls, it is not unusual for further lobes to become emphysematous fairly soon after the operation.

Necrotizing enterocolitis

This condition carries a mortality as high as 50 per cent in most series. It affects up to 8 per cent of patients in special care units, and is characterized by abdominal distension with ileus, blood in the stools and a typical X-ray appearance of gas in the bowel wall. This last—pneumatosis intestinalis—is often preceded by thickening of the bowel wall by oedema. The portal venous system within the liver may be outlined by gas; 50 per cent of the patients have a Gram-negative septicaemia (Fig. 4.11).

There has been a considerable increase in the incidence of necrotizing enterocolitis in recent years. The cause of this is uncertain, but may be related to improved resuscitation in low birth weight infants who have suffered intra- or postnatal asphyxia. Many of these babies would have died, but now survive to suffer the consequences of ischaemic damage to organs such as the gut. Asphyxia certainly causes diversion of blood flow from the gut by up to 85 per cent to preserve the flow to other more vital organs such as the brain and the heart. It has been shown in the experimental animal that such haemodynamic changes can result in necrosis in the gut, causing perforations and peritonitis.

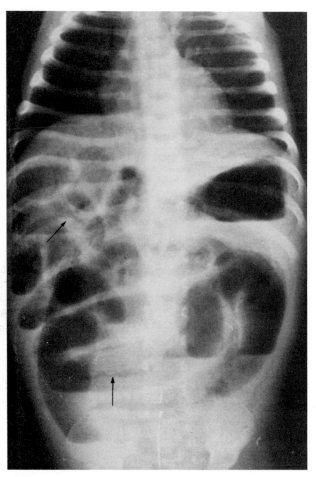

Fig. 4.11 Necrotizing enterocolitis. Erect X-ray showing distended loops of bowel, with fluid levels, intramural gas and gas in the portal venous system.

Most babies with necrotizing enterocolitis have a history of birth asphyxia and many have recovered from hyaline membrane disease. Approximately 60 per cent of cases have had umbilical artery or venous catheterization. Other factors may also operate, such as Gram-negative bacterial infections, milk formula as opposed to breast feeding and possible damage to gut mucosa from hyperosmolar feeds.

The babies must start a regimen of intravenous feeding and of nasogastric suction, and any umbilical catheters must be removed. The cardiovascular system must be closely monitored and if the peripheral circulation is poor, blood or plasma should be transfused. Gentamicin or similar antibiotic should be given. These babies often require total intravenous nutrition (see p. 166).

At any stage, surgical intervention may be necessary if it is possible that perforation has occurred as suggested by fluid or free gas in the abdominal X-ray.

Occasionally, respiratory failure may ensue and this is especially likely postoperatively.

After the acute stage is over, fibrotic healing causing bowel strictures may occur, again bringing the patient to the operating theatre.

Urogenital abnormalities

The commonest lesions causing urinary tract obstructions in the neonate are pelvic hydronephrosis and posterior urethral valves.

The cause of hydronephrosis is not fully understood but considerable damage to the renal parenchyma may result. The commonest presenting symptoms are a palpable abdominal mass and non-specific symptoms such as failure to thrive associated with urinary tract infections. Diagnosis is confirmed radiologically, and surgery usually consists of pyeloureteroplasty. The babies occasionally have severe electrolyte and fluid disturbances.

Urethral valves

Posterior urethral valves which cause obstruction in the neonate usually present because of uraemia, acidaemia and the toxic effects of severe urinary infection. Vomiting and failure to thrive are common presenting symptoms; in a severe case, cardiorespiratory collapse may occur following a vicious circle of vomiting, dehydration, reduced renal function, acidosis and fall in cardiac output. Abnormalities of micturition may go unnoticed.

The valves, which may be thick and rigid, tend to pass downwards and laterally, extending around the lumen of the urethra, and fuse together at a lower level. Catheterization and instrumentation are easily carried out, but the valve cusps obstruct the flow of urine. The obstruction to urine flow can have a very severe effect on the developing urinary tract, often before birth. The long-term prognosis must depend on the degree of renal damage; in one series, 22 of 54 boys presenting within 3 months of age died. The amount of irreversible kidney damage cannot be assessed from the initial degree of uraemia, which is caused also by dehydration, obstruction to urine flow and infection in a very sick baby.

Initial treatment must include fluids intravenously for dehydration, sodium bicarbonate to correct acidosis, antibiotics and urinary catheterization. Surgery is indicated only when metabolic correction has taken place. Definitive diagnosis requires radiography (retrograde cystogram). The great majority of urethral valves may be destroyed by fulguration throughout their length, using a cystoscope. When the instrument cannot be passed through a small anterior urethra, a urethrostomy in the perineum is created to enable the cystoscope to enter the posterior urethra.

Anaesthesia should follow the basic principles for neonatal patients; if adequate medical treatment has been carried out initially, then no additional problems should ensue. After relief of the obstruction, a large fluid intake may be required, depending on the urine output and its osmolality. Up to 1 litre of fluid may be required over the first 12 hours postoperatively in severe cases. Potassium supplements are often necessary for these cases, though serum electrolyte values are used as a guide for intravenous doses of potassium.

Prune belly syndrome

The prune belly syndrome (Fig. 4.12), which involves defective muscularization of the anterior abdominal wall and the urinary tract, is only seen in its full extent in males. The full syndrome is a complex with several developmental errors. The severity of the muscular defect varies and may involve one or both sides of the abdominal wall. The skin over the abdomen is classically wrinkled like a prune, though it may merely have abnormal transverse creases. The costal margin is flared and the sternum is unusually prominent. The upper parts of the recti and the oblique muscles of the abdomen are usually present.

Abnormalities of the gastrointestinal tract may include volvulus and intestinal obstruction, but changes in the genitourinary system are commonly seen and their severity is proportional to the deficiency of the abdominal musculature. The bladder is large and the urachus patent as far as the umbilicus. The ureters are dilated and the pelves of the kidneys may be similarly affected; the degree of dysfunction depends on the back-pressure effect of the urine and subsequent urinary tract infection. The testes are always undescended.

These babies may have renal failure, acidosis and dehydration and may also be septicaemic. Because of the absent abdominal musculature, they may have reduced pulmonary function, with an inability to cough and clear the chest of secretions.

Surgery is designed to restore function of the urinary tract, to improve emptying of the bladder and to preserve or improve renal function.

The anaesthetist must take into account the possibility that renal function may be impaired, so care must be taken with those drugs known to be excreted in the urine. There is usually a history of repeated chest infections, and any infection of the chest or urinary tract should be vigorously treated preoperatively. The babies should be managed during induction as if the stomach were full, because of the danger of regurgitation of gastric contents. The neonate is intubated awake, and controlled ventilation is maintained *without* the use of relaxants because the abdomen is very lax anyway. Postoperatively, hypoventilation and a reduced coughing mechanism may cause sputum retention and respiratory failure. Extubation takes place only when the baby is fully awake and moving vigorously.

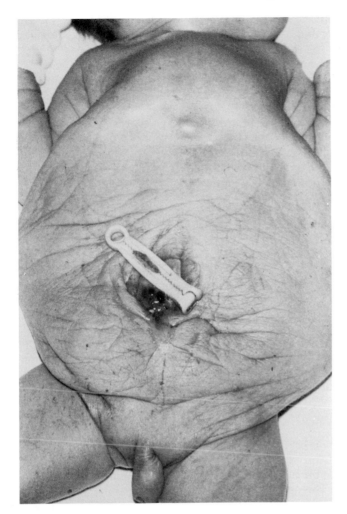

Fig. 4.12 The prune belly syndrome.

Bladder exstrophy

This serious congenital malformation affects approximately 1 in 20 000 babies: three times as many males as females. The mucosa of the bladder is laid open and the ureteric orifices are visible. The size of the exstrophy varies and sometimes the surface area of the mucosa is the same as that of a normal bladder. There is complete epispadias. As the mucosa of the bladder continues to be exposed, it becomes hyperaemic, friable and infected. Hydroureteronephrosis may develop because of oedema and later fibrosis which affect the ureteric orifices, causing obstruction to urine outflow.

Definitive surgical treatment is usually undertaken in the neonate before infection and secondary ureteric problems arise and while the bladder is still thin-walled and flexible. The open bladder exstrophy, if left, may predispose to carcinoma. The results of closure do not necessarily indicate that full continence and a normal upper urinary tract can be expected.

The operation involves major surgery, starting with the patient prone for bilateral osteotomies of the iliac bones after which the baby is positioned supine for formal mobilization and closure of the bladder. The pelvic osteotomies enable the pubes to be apposed and closure of the urethra to be attempted. Heavy blood loss may be expected and two good intravenous lines should be established, one of which could be central in the internal jugular vein. Hypotensive anaesthesia, so useful for this operation in older children, is rarely necessary in the neonate. Full monitoring should include oesophageal stethoscope and blood pressure cuff. Care should be taken to prevent heat loss during the long operation, particularly at the stage of turning from the prone to supine positions. The endotracheal tube and intravenous lines should be very well secured to prevent accidental dislodgement during turning of the baby. While the baby is prone, pads under the pelvis and chest prevent pressure on the inferior vena cava which would increase bleeding and also decrease cardiac output.

Anaesthesia for neuroradiology and neurosurgery

The principles of anaesthesia for neuroradiological investigation and neurosurgery in neonates do not differ greatly from those in adults. All patients need very careful neurological assessment preoperatively.

Cerebral blood flow

Cerebral blood flow is normally regulated automatically to match cerebral metabolism. Decreased oxygenation of arterial blood results in an increased rate of blood flow to the brain so that tissue oxygen tension is maintained at near normal levels. This autoregulation operates throughout a wide range of systemic blood pressure (60–180 mmHg in the adult) and even as low as 45–50 mmHg in the newborn infant. Cerebral blood flow increases with increasing arterial carbon dioxide tension ($Paco_2$) between 20 and 80 mmHg: hypocapnia tends to modify the effects of agents that increase cerebral blood flow. Damaged areas of brain, such as occur with trauma, infarction or in the region of arteriovenous malformations and tumours, lose their autoregulation so the circulation in these areas varies passively with blood pressure. If the $Paco_2$ rises and normal cerebral vessels dilate, blood is diverted from abnormal to healthy areas (intracerebral steal syndrome). The inverse intracerebral steal syndrome is seen when normally reactive cerebral vessels constrict.

The total volume of the intracranial contents cannot alter within the rigid skull of the adult, though compensatory decreases (or increases) may take place within the three constituents: brain, blood and cerebrospinal fluid (CSF). A slowly expanding space-occupying lesion will displace CSF and venous blood, so intracranial pressure (ICP) rises very slowly until no more compensation is possible. Any small increase in volume above this will cause a very large increase in ICP with severe symptoms. A neonatal skull has a capacity to expand not seen with the rigid adult skull and increasing head circumference is the main sign of hydrocephalus, preceding symptoms of raised ICP (vomiting, irritability, seizures or severe lethargy).

All inhalational anaesthetic agents increase cerebral blood flow, as does ketamine, although intravenous induction agents, barbiturates and drugs which depress neuronal activity tend to decrease it. Halothane, like all inhalational anaesthetic agents, increases cerebral blood flow and thus intracranial pressure. The effect is minimal if low doses of halothane are used, and is not seen if hyperventilation is employed. This makes halothane combined with mild hyperventilation a very useful technique for neonatal neurosurgical anaesthesia.

Anaesthesia for neuroradiology

General anaesthesia is invariably required for major neuroradiological investigations because of the need for immobility and the prolonged discomfort involved.

In addition to the problems of anaesthetizing a neonate, there are those associated with working in the X-ray department. The commonest problem is a lack of facilities for keeping the baby warm, but this can be overcome with warm coverings and a draught-free environment. There is the possibility of static electricity or electrical sparks, so cyclopropane should be avoided and, because of the risk of radiation, protective aprons must be worn by the staff. Fewer invasive investigations have been necessary since the advent of the computerized axial tomography (CAT) scanner.

CAT scan

Neonates do not need anaesthesia for CAT scanning as restraint with a blanket will immobilize the infant for the procedure. Occasionally, intubation is necessary for airway security in patients who are having fits or are comatose or in respiratory failure.

Lumbar air encephalography

This is rarely necessary nowadays but is still needed for pituitary fossa lesions and for confirmation of the site of obstruction to the flow of CSF if this is not obvious from the CAT scan.

As for all neuroradiological and neurosurgical anaesthesia, only atropine is given for premedication. Increased steroid cover is necessary if the patient has been given dexamethasone for treatment of any intracranial problem. The patient is intubated awake using a non-kinking type of tube such as the Magill flexometallic tube, introduced with a rigid stilette. This tube must be very firmly fixed because the radiological examination requires tilting and somersaulting of the patient, during which accidental extubation may occur.

A relaxant technique using tubocurarine and controlled ventilation is necessary for the neonate, though older babies may be allowed to breathe spontaneously. The limbs are wrapped in foil and as much of the baby as possible is swaddled in warm coverings. The oesophageal stethoscope, ECG and blood pressure cuff should be used to monitor the patient's condition.

Respiratory signs of rising ICP will be lost with controlled ventilation so, as air is injected, careful monitoring of cardiovascular signs, such as rising pulse and blood pressure, is necessary. It is possible that an acute rise in ICP may cause coning of the brain stem, with respiratory and cardiovascular signs; the pulse rate will slow and a spontaneously breathing patient will become apnoeic. Immediate steps must be taken to relieve the ICP and osmotic diuretics such as mannitol $2 \, g \cdot kg^{-1}$ and an urgent ventricular tap may be necessary.

The anaesthetic T-piece is an ideal circuit for use in the X-ray department, as a long lead for fresh gas flow and a long expiratory limb do not alter the function of the circuit but help the anaesthetist during moving of the patient.

After reversal of any neuromuscular block, the patient is extubated when fully awake and returned as soon as possible to the recovery area where postoperative neurological assessment can begin.

Myelography

Myelography is performed for investigation of spinal cord injuries at birth, cord compressions and for dysraphic lesions of the cord.

Diastematomyelia is a fissure or cleft of the spinal cord in the lumbar region, caused by transfixion of the neural tissue by a bony septum. This prevents normal ascent of the cord in the vertebral canal as the child grows and, because the cord is tethered in the lumbar region, there will be progressive neurological damage. Cutaneous haemangiomata, a lipoma or a tuft of hair may overlie the site of the spinal defect.

During the X-ray examination there is a need for many changes in position of the patient, including marked flexion of the head, and a flexible reinforced endotracheal tube is therefore recommended. If the investigation includes the cervical spine, a radiolucent tube must be used; a plain Portex tube is suitable.

Premedication is with atropine and awake intubation carried out after preoxygenation. Intubation difficulties are occasionally encountered, as lesions of the cervical spine which need investigation may be associated with conditions such as the Klippel–Feil syndrome (p. 190).

Cisternal air myelograms are rarely performed nowadays and there are several reports of air embolism in the literature. Metrizamide, the radio-opaque contrast medium used for myelography, causes seizures if it is allowed to track up into the head. The contrast medium is only given during screening and about 5 ml is used for a neonate. The threshold for seizures is markedly reduced if the patient receives phenothiazines, so these should be avoided.

Vital signs should be monitored using an oesophageal stethoscope and a blood pressure cuff. The most satisfactory anaesthetic technique involves a relaxant, controlled ventilation with oxygen, nitrous oxide and incremental halothane (0.25–0.5 per cent). Hypotension may occur during tilting of the patient.

Great care should be taken to prevent contrast medium from draining into the head, so a head-up posture is necessary postoperatively. It is perhaps wisest to give phenobarbitone 2 mg·kg⁻¹ intramuscularly after the investigation as a precaution against seizures.

Angiography

Carotid angiograms are performed for suspected vascular malformations and arteriovenous malformations and tumours (rare in the neonatal period). Arteriovenous malformations may present with cardiac failure, and a bruit over the head will be audible. Fits will need to be controlled with specific agents.

Premedication is with atropine, and awake intubation is carried out after preoxygenation. Ventilation, which needs to be controlled for neonatal anaesthesia, is also an advantage for cerebral arteriography. A flexible reinforced endotracheal tube is used. If the patient is ventilated to a $Paco_2$ of 4 kPa (30 mmHg), normal vessels are constricted, which improves the definition of abnormal vessels. The dose of contrast medium must not exceed 4 ml·kg⁻¹ body weight. Allergic reactions to contrast medium are relatively common and cause death in 1 in 40 000 cases. The contrast is hypertonic and causes a biphasic problem for the circulation: initial volume overload, followed by dehydration after an osmotic diuresis. Contrast media may also interfere with the clotting mechanism in which platelets are consumed. It is possible for a baby to lose 10 per cent of the circulating blood volume during a carotid angiogram, and fluid overload is possible as the result of excessive flushing of the artery with saline.

Anaesthesia for neurosurgery

Neurosurgery in the neonatal period usually involves operations for developmental anomalies in the spine and cranium, for hydrocephalus or for extradural and subdural haematomas. Most operations for tumours, craniosynostosis or vascular lesions tend to fall into this age group.

Myelomeningocele

Myelomeningocele occurs in 1–4 infants per 1000 live births, though encephalocele is much less common (1 in 5000). The measurement of α-fetoprotein concentrations in the amniotic fluid has made possible the antenatal recognition of severe open neural tube anomalies and possible termination of the pregnancy. The maternal serum α-fetoprotein may also be elevated in pregnancy when the fetus has an open neural tube anomaly.

After 1952, when it became possible to relieve hydrocephalus by shunt operations, a period of aggressive surgery for myelomeningocele followed in which closure of the back lesion was one of the most common emergency neonatal operations. Because of the very large numbers of badly deformed children who survived as a result of this policy, many centres now try to restrict surgical treatment at birth to those babies whose handicap later in life will be minimal. Back closure is carried out in these babies within 24–36 hours of life because to delay increases the chances of wound infection and meningitis. However, some untreated babies survive and in these back closure must be considered at some stage on humanitarian grounds.

Eighty per cent of babies with myelomeningocele or encephalocele develop hydrocephalus with the Arnold–Chiari malformation (downward displacement of the pons and medulla and protrusion of the cerebellar vermis through the foramen magnum) and aqueduct stenosis. Occasionally, patients with the Arnold–Chiari malformation develop stridor as hydrocephalus progresses. This is possibly caused by traction on the vagus nerve in the posterior cranial fossa. Usually the stridor disappears after insertion of a shunt or occipital craniectomy.

Occipital encephalocele is very commonly associated with other abnormalities such as Klippel–Feil syndrome (webbing of the neck and cervical vertebral synostosis), micrognathia and cleft palate. Such patients may be very difficult to intubate. If the neural damage is very extensive and possibly involving autonomic functions in the midbrain, then surgery is usually withheld.

Surgery involves excision of the sac and preservation of the neural elements, then closure of the defect with fascial flaps and skin coverage. In the past, a very large defect needed a rotation flap of skin for cover.

Preoperatively the lesion is covered with sterile gauze, blood is crossmatched, and atropine and vitamin K (1 mg) are given as premedication. Awake intubation is performed using a plain or flexometallic endotracheal tube with the patient on his side to minimize damage to the myelomeningocele or encephalocele. An assistant presses the shoulders back and supports the head in an optimum position for laryngoscopy. An alternative is to support the baby's back on a 'head ring' to protect the lesion from pressure while the baby is intubated in the usual supine position.

For surgery, the infant is positioned prone, usually with pads supporting the chest and pelvis so that the abdomen remains free from external pressure and inferior vena caval obstruction is avoided. Any venous obstruction will greatly increase bleeding from the wound. When the patient is in the prone position, care must be taken to protect the eyes—which should be taped down after chloramphenicol eye ointment has been inserted. In certain conditions such as gross hydrocephalus or hypertelorism, the eyes may be very difficult to close and tarsorrhaphy is occasionally necessary.

Anaesthesia is usually maintained with oxygen, nitrous oxide and halothane up to 0.5 per cent with controlled ventilation. Controlled ventilation is especially necessary for neonates operated on in the prone position with pressure on the chest. Relaxants may be used if the surgeon does not need to use a nerve stimulator to confirm the position of nerve roots. The vital signs are monitored using an oesophageal stethoscope, ECG, blood pressure cuff and rectal temperature probe.

Maintenance of normal body temperature, which is so important in paediatric anaesthesia, is very difficult indeed in neurosurgery. Surgeons should be discouraged from using cold, wet drapes. The limbs and trunk must be wrapped in foil and as much contact as possible obtained between the baby and the heating pad. It is possible to put the support pads beneath the heating pad rather than between it and the baby. With most cases of occipital encephalocele some temperature fall during surgery is inevitable

A further difficulty is the measurement of blood loss since this is mixed with unknown quantities of CSF and saline used for irrigation. The need for transfusion is assessed not only by estimation of blood loss, but also by changes in the patient's vital signs, including the state of the peripheral circulation, pulse rate and blood pressure. As a rule blood is needed for encephalocele, but not for myelomeningocele. In infants the suboccipital bone is very vascular. Surgery for occipital encephalocele involves a risk of air embolism because the suboccipital bones are exposed. Careful monitoring with an oesophageal stethoscope and ECG should give warning of this potentially disastrous complication. The surgeons may also be in a position to warn the anaesthetist. Venous distension, to discourage the passage of the air into the heart, is then possible by applying pressure to the reservoir bag of the anaesthetic T-piece.

For spinal surgery in cases of diastematomyelia the general anaesthesia principles described for excision of myelomeningocele also apply. Blood loss may be expected to exceed 10 per cent of the blood volume and this must be replaced. Careful positioning of the chest and pelvis on pads will minimize venous bleeding from the edges of vertebrae.

Hydrocephalus

A large section of neurosurgery in the neonate is carried out for hydrocephalus. The abnormal accumulation of CSF within the head is usually obstructive due to blockage of the fluid pathway. Communicating hydrocephalus with an open CSF pathway into the subarachnoid space may occur after meningitis. Non-communicating hydrocephalus is due to obstruction of the fluid pathway proximal to the subarachnoid space, such as aqueduct stenosis, or Arnold–Chiari syndrome.

Hydrocephalus is very commonly associated with myelomeningocele. The combined defect is present in 3 per 1000 live births. The excess CSF causes rapid dilatation of the ventricles, destroying the brain and producing enlargement of the cranium. The earliest sign is one of increasing head circumference, which is routinely measured in all babies following operation for myelomeningocele. Bulging fontanelle, the 'setting sun' sign of the eyes and increased spasticity of the limbs are all later signs. Papilloedema is rare because of the capacity for the infant skull to dilate. Ten per cent of these children will grow up to be very retarded.

Surgical treatment involves the use of a low pressure valve (such as the Spitz–Holter) draining CSF from the ventricle to the right atrium, to the pleural cavity or to the peritoneum for cases for non-communicating hydrocephalus. For communicating hydrocephalus a shunt is inserted from the lumbar subarachnoid space to the peritoneum. If the CSF is infected, surgery must be delayed because the valve will become colonized.

The most important neonatal sign of raised intracranial pressure is the tendency to apnoeic attacks. Such patients need to be intubated, ventilated and a ventricular tap performed. Cardiovascular signs such as bradycardia are also indicative of raised ICP.

Premedication is with atropine, and after preoxygenation awake intubation is performed with a flexible tube. Difficulties with intubation associated with a very large head may be avoided if the patient's trunk is placed on a pillow so that the head is in neutral position. Controlled ventilation is established, preferably using a relaxant/nitrous oxide/oxygen technique and the baby is monitored with oesophageal stethoscope, ECG and blood pressure cuff. Cardiovascular instability may occur at any time and is related to changes in ICP, especially hypotension at the time of CSF tap if the ICP and systemic blood pressure were previously raised. It is necessary to ventilate the patient with 100 per cent oxygen at this stage. At the moment that the internal jugular vein is opened for insertion of the catheter, positive pressure on the reservoir bag of the T-piece will raise the venous pressure and prevent air embolism. Ventriculoatrial shunts are usually inserted under X-ray control so that the distal catheter is seen to lie in the right atrium. The ECG may also be used as a guide to positioning the atrial end of the shunt. The shunt tubing is filled with hypertonic saline and attached to the left arm ECG lead. As the tip approaches the right atrium, the P-waves grow taller and when in the correct position the P-waves become small again and biphasic.

An anaesthetic technique involving spontaneous ventilation with halothane is acceptable for older babies and has the advantage of preserving respiratory signs of changing intracranial pressure.

The patient should be wide awake before extubation and be returned to the intensive care unit for neurological assessment postoperatively. Though blood is always cross-matched for this operation it is very rarely used. Phenobarbitone 1 mg·kg^{-1} intramuscularly 6-hourly and codeine phosphate 1 mg·kg^{-1} intramuscularly 6-hourly are prescribed for sedation postoperatively, but this should very rarely be needed in the neonatal period.

Other conditions

Other neurosurgical conditions which may require surgery in the neonate include intracranial haematomas and craniosynostosis (premature fusion of the cranial sutures, leading to deformities and mental retardation). Massive blood loss may be a feature of these operations, though anaesthesia follows the general pattern of that for neurosurgery in the neonate. Blood loss may be particularly large with craniectomy for craniosynostosis, and direct measurement of arterial pressure is useful so that the systolic blood pressure can be reduced to the range 50–60 mmHg using an increased halothane concentration and controlled ventilation. Induced hypotension with trimetaphan or sodium nitroprusside is not necessary in the neonate. After craniectomy, babies may lose at least 10 per cent of the blood volume into a drain or into the head bandages.

Surgery in the sitting position is very rare indeed in the neonatal period, though it is widely used for posterior fossa exploration and cervical surgery in the older child. However, the neonatal anaesthetist must be aware of the dangers of air embolism in any neurosurgical procedure where the head may be higher than the trunk.

Anaesthesia for cardiac surgery

The incidence of major congenital heart disease is estimated at 6–8 per 1000 live births. Without treatment, approximately 50 per cent of these children will die in the first year of life, one-third of the deaths occurring in the first 3 months of life. Neonates with congenital heart disease may present as emergencies because of the effects of the cardiac anomaly itself, because of the effects of prematurity or because of the presence of other major congenital abnormalities. Of the coincident defects, renal abnormalities are the most common, though cleft palate, tracheo-oesophageal fistula, abdominal malformations and other defects also occur.

Ventricular septal defect is the commonest congenital cardiac anomaly, with an incidence of 2 per 1000 live births, though at least three-quarters of these defects will close spontaneously. Patent ductus arteriosus, pulmonary stenosis and atrial septal defect have incidences of 0.5–0.7 per 1000 live births. Transposition of the great arteries, though the commonest cardiac anomaly to cause cyanosis in the newborn, is an even rarer lesion, having a similar incidence to aortic stenosis, coarctation of the aorta and Fallot's tetralogy (0.3 per 1000 live births). Total anomalous pulmonary venous drainage, although having an incidence of only 0.1 per 1000 live births, is an extremely serious lesion in the newborn, often requiring emergency surgery because of severe hypoxia and congestive cardiac failure.

Though open heart operations in the first month of life are still associated with a high overall mortality (Table 4.2), two points must be borne in mind.

Table 4.2 Open heart operations in infancy (Great Ormond Street) 1971–1979

Age (months)	Number	Deaths
0– 1	85	43 (51%)
1– 6	197	50 (25%)
6–12	153	22 (14%)

First, these operations are carried out on sick babies who would all certainly die without treatment. Second, many of the babies have complex, multiple lesions. If these are excluded, the mortality of the remainder is seen to be considerably lower (Table 4.3).

Table 4.3 Neonatal open heart operations (Great Ormond Street) 1971–1979

	Number	Deaths
Simple lesions (VSD, PS, AS, TGA)	24	6 (25%)
Complex lesions (TAPVD, truncus arteriosus, pulmonary atresia, complex AS, VSD and TGA, etc.)	61	37 (61%)
Total	85	43 (51%)

AS, aortic stenosis;   PS, pulmonary stenosis;   TAPVD, total anomalous pulmonary venous drainage;   TGA, transposition of the great arteries;   VSD, ventricular septal defect.

Preoperative management

Severe congenital cardiac anomalies in the newborn can be classified into three main categories.

1. Those which cause cardiac failure: ventricular septal defect, patent ductus arteriosus, aortic stenosis, coarctation of the aorta.
2. Those which cause cyanosis: pulmonary atresia, Fallot's tetralogy (rarely cyanosed in the neonatal period), tricuspid atresia and single ventricle with pulmonary stenosis.
3. Those which cause failure and cyanosis: transposition of the great arteries, truncus arteriosus, total anomalous pulmonary venous drainage.

Babies in cardiac failure usually develop severe hypoxaemia and acidosis, often complicated by hypoglycaemia or hypocalcaemia. They may require ventilatory support if they are in respiratory failure, inotropic support if cardiac output is low, diuretics if overhydrated and intravenous fluids if dry.

Immediate assessment should include measurement of blood sugar, calcium and electrolyte levels, and arterial blood gas and acid–base analysis. Fifty per cent dextrose should be given intravenously ($0.2\,ml\cdot kg^{-1}$) if the blood sugar falls below $2\,mmol\cdot l^{-1}$ in a full-term neonate or $1.5\,mmol\cdot l^{-1}$ in a premature neonate. If the serum calcium is less than $2.0\,mmol\cdot l^{-1}$, intravenous 20 per cent calcium gluconate should be given ($1\,ml\cdot kg^{-1}$). ECG and body temperature should be monitored, and the baby nursed in a suitably warm environment.

Diagnostic procedures

Cardiac catheterization and angiocardiography are still required to substantiate the diagnosis in most neonates with suspected congenital heart disease. However, many lesions are now capable of elucidation by real time, two-dimensional echocardiography. In the future this may either completely replace catheterization and angiography or at least significantly reduce their use. These procedures are usually carried out without general anaesthesia, and sedation is often unnecessary in the newborn baby. After the first few days of life, a sedative intramuscular injection of pethidine compound up to $0.05\,ml\cdot kg^{-1}$ body weight is usually given half an hour prior to catheterization (1 ml pethidine compound contains 25 mg pethidine, 6.25 mg chlorpromazine and 6.25 mg promethazine). This is half the dose used in older infants. Should any additional sedation be required during the investigation, diazepam $0.1 \, mg \cdot kg^{-1}$ may be injected through the cardiac catheter. If general anaesthesia is considered essential, endotracheal intubation should be performed and a nitrous oxide/oxygen mixture administered using full muscle relaxation (pancuronium $0.04 \, mg \cdot kg^{-1}$ or tubocurarine $0.2 \, mg \cdot kg^{-1}$) and controlled ventilation of the lungs. It is essential to monitor inspired oxygen concentration. It is impossible to calculate shunts if the oxygen saturation of the venous blood is too high.

The newborn baby, if premature, is especially susceptible to heat loss, and steps should be taken to avoid hypothermia. The temperature of the room should not be less than 24°C, the baby should be swathed in warm clothing and, if possible, be placed on a radiolucent heating pad. Wrapping the head and limbs in aluminium foil also helps to reduce heat loss.

In small infants, excessive amounts of blood can easily be removed during diagnostic sampling unless oximetry is carried out in a sterilized cuvette from which the sample can be returned to the patient. The blood volume in the neonate is approximately $85 \, ml \cdot kg^{-1}$ body weight and loss of more than 10 per cent of this usually requires replacement. Blood should be cross-matched at the start of the procedure.

Other hazards of cardiac catheterization are rare. They include dysrhythmias, occasional perforation of the heart and hypotension. The last is commonly related to hypovolaemia or dysrhythmia resulting from intracardiac manipulation of the catheter. Systemic hypotension may lead to increase in any right-to-left shunting and intense hypoxia. Hypoxaemia itself may increase pulmonary vascular resistance and thus create a vicious circle of events. Contrast medium is hypertonic and may cause fluid retention.

The pericatheter mortality in the first month of life is probably around 10 per cent but it is difficult to separate the hazards of the investigation from those of the cardiac lesion itself.

'Open heart' procedures

General principles

'Open heart' surgery in infancy has developed greatly in the last 10 years, with falling mortality (Fig. 4.13). This is due to advances in equipment and techniques, as well as to improved preoperative diagnosis. Better oxygenators are now available, of both the bubble and membrane type, with 'priming volume' reduced to 750–1000 ml. Improved intracardiac cannulae and suckers cause less red cell damage, and the use of blood filters has reduced platelet–fibrin aggregation with its risk of embolization. The technique of surface cooling to 26–28°C prior to sternotomy has made ventricular fibrillation in the immediate prebypass period a less worrying problem, and is said to produce more even 'core cooling' than the conventional blood stream method. The use of profound hypothermia by blood stream cooling on bypass to temperatures of 18–20°C allows the surgeon to carry out the intracardiac repair on a bloodless motionless heart during periods of up to 60 minutes' circulatory arrest, and reduces the time on bypass. Cooling to

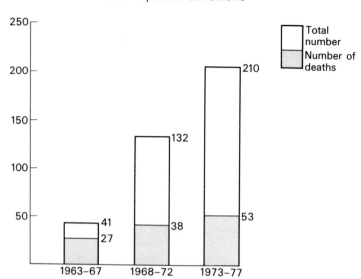

Fig. 4.13 Open heart surgery in the first year of life at the Hospital for Sick Children, Great Ormond Street, 1963–1977. (Courtesy of J. Stark)

much lower temperatures (4–6°C) has been advocated recently, though this technique has not yet been fully evaluated.

Perfusion technique in neonates

Until recently, fresh heparinized blood was chosen to prime the bypass for neonatal surgery because of the risk of coagulation disorders following the use of stored blood, and because of the metabolic alkalosis which follows the transfusion of citrated blood. Fresh blood is difficult to obtain, especially in an emergency, but the freshest stored blood obtainable should be used. Haemodilution should not lower the haematocrit below 30 per cent because the newborn neonate has difficulty in excreting a large fluid load. Haemodilution does, however, improve the flow characteristics of the perfusate, especially at low temperatures, and improves postperfusion urine flow; 20 mg heparin, 3 ml of 20 per cent calcium chloride and 80 mmol sodium bicarbonate are added to each unit of blood primed. Mannitol ($0.5\,g\cdot kg^{-1}$) may be added to improve urine output, and methylprendisolone sodium succinate (SoluMedrone) ($30\,mg\cdot kg^{-1}$) to stabilize membranes. Some also add albumin to increase the osmotic pressure of the prime. Bypass flow rate is calculated at $2.4\,l\cdot m^{-2}$ per minute, though lower flows are used during hypothermia.

Technique of surface cooling

The anaesthetized infant is placed on a water blanket through which ice-cold water is circulating, and small ice-filled plastic bags are packed around and under the body (Fig. 4.14). Care should be taken to avoid placing icebags directly over the precordium because of the risk of ventricular fibrillation, or on the extremities of limbs or in the area of the kidneys, as this may reduce renal blood flow. The bags should be moved occasionally to avoid thermal damage to the skin from the ice.

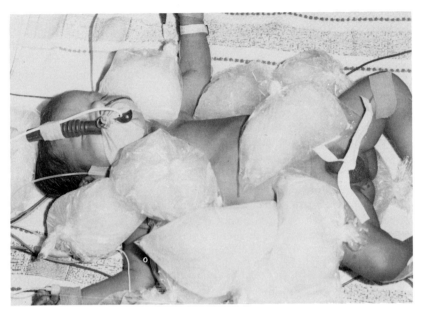

Fig. 4.14   The position of icebags for surface cooling.

While cooling is taking place, the ECG, nasopharyngeal and oesophageal temperatures should be monitored, and arterial and central venous lines, if not already in place, should be inserted. Blood pressure should be monitored with a Doppler flowmeter until direct arterial pressure monitoring is established. Shivering and vasoconstriction should be prevented by full muscle relaxation together with the addition of small doses of chlorpromazine ($0.5\,mg\cdot kg^{-1}$). As the metabolic rate falls with falling temperature, carbon dioxide production decreases and 2.5–5 per cent carbon dioxide should be added to the inspired gas mixture once the nasopharyngeal temperature reaches 34°C, because this improves cerebral perfusion and helps to avoid intense vasoconstriction. Blood gases and serum potassium should be checked regularly during cooling. Supplements of potassium are frequently required at this stage as potassium may move into the cells. Arterial carbon dioxide tension (corrected for the low temperature of the blood sample) should be kept above 6 kPa (45 mmHg) and serum potassium should not be allowed to fall below $3\,mmol\cdot l^{-1}$.

Active cooling is discontinued once the nasopharyngeal temperature has reached 26–28°C. Icebags are removed, the infant is carefully dried and surgery commenced. Any sudden movements of the baby's position at this stage can cause ventricular fibrillation. Temperature usually drifts down 2°C further.

Anaesthetic management

Premedication.   Neonates are given atropine (0.15–0.2 mg) either alone or with pethidine compound in reduced dosage (0.05 mg·kg^{-1}) 1 hour pre-operatively.

Before bypass.   ECG, precordial heartbeat and Doppler blood pressure should be monitored before induction of anaesthesia. The sickest babies and those in the first week or two of life may be intubated awake without difficulty, and some may already have required intubation before reaching the operating theatre. In older neonates, especially if vigorous, it may be wiser to intubate under light general anaesthesia and muscle relaxation. Halothane is potentially dangerous at this stage because of the risk of hypotension and must be used with extreme caution. It is completely contraindicated in infants with left ventricular outflow tract obstruction, where hypotension and ventricular fibrillation occur very readily and where the nitrous oxide/oxygen/muscle relaxant technique is safer. An endotracheal tube of 2.5 or 3.0 mm internal diameter is passed and either the oral or nasal route can be used. The former is usually easier and quicker, and less likely to cause hypoxia, but will have to be changed at the end of the operation as a nasal tube can be secured more satisfactorily for postoperative care. It is important to make sure there is air entry to both lungs after intubation, as it is quite easy to intubate either main bronchus.

Arterial, central venous and peripheral venous lines can usually be inserted percutaneously. It is wise to establish a venous line as soon as possible so that resuscitative drugs can be given if required. The arterial line is preferably inserted into a radial artery and the central venous line into the right internal jugular vein by the technique described by English *et al.* (1964). The head is turned away from the side to be cannulated and a small sandbag is placed under the shoulders. A skin incision is made over the medial border of the sternomastoid muscle, just lateral to the carotid artery and half-way between the mastoid process and the sternoclavicular joint. The cannula is advanced downwards and laterally in the direction of the nipple. It should enter the internal jugular vein soon after passing through the substance of the sternomastoid muscle. Pressure over the liver by an assistant helps to fill the vein and makes cannulation easier. In the presence of a left superior vena cava it may be necessary to cannulate the left internal jugular vein as well. Major complications of cannulation of the radial artery are rare in children—provided a fine (22 s.w.g. for neonates) cannula is used—possibly because the arterial wall is healthier, or because there is a better collateral blood supply. Internal jugular cannulation is not free from hazard, particularly from puncture of the carotid artery with haematoma formation or from pneumothorax. The advantages are generally felt to outweigh the risks involved, which may be minimized if the tip of the needle is kept well above the thoracic inlet. It is seldom possible to advance a percutaneous cannula centrally from the antecubital fossa in infants. If venous or aterial cannulation fails, it may be necessary to cut down onto a limb vessel. Oesophageal and nasopharyngeal or rectal temperatures should also be monitored, the former reflecting blood temperature and the latter core temperature. EEG with the cerebral function monitor is recommended to ensure that cerebral function is adequately depressed by the hypothermia before perfusion is stopped. Intermittent positive pressure ventilation (IPPV) is continued with 50 per cent nitrous oxide/oxygen as the basic anaesthetic, and pancuronium 0.1–0.15 mg·kg^{-1} for muscle relaxation. The inspired gas should be warmed and humidified. Narcotic supplements such as morphine (up to 0.5 mg·kg^{-1} after test dose) may be used if the cardiovascular system is stable. A supply of emergency drugs should be immediately available, including 8.4 per cent sodium bicarbonate and 20 per cent calcium chloride. A urinary catheter is inserted and urine output recorded regularly. Heparin 3 mg·kg^{-1} is given prior to insertion of the aortic cannula, and it is wise to check the level of heparinization by the activated coagulation time (ACT). Additional muscle relaxant should be given at least 10 minutes before commencement of bypass to allow time for it to be fixed at the neuromuscular end-plate, and an incremental dose of narcotic may be required at this stage.

During bypass.   It is not necessary to ventilate the lungs during bypass, and opinions vary as to what gas mixture they should contain at this time. Some fill them with inert gas such as helium, but many leave them gently distended with oxygen or air at about 5 cmH$_2$O. Heparinization should be checked every 30 minutes using the ACT, but since relatively large amounts of heparin are added to the perfusate during priming, incremental doses of heparin are virtually never required.

Myocardial function is preserved during bypass by the use of ice-cold cardioplegic solution injected into the aortic root and hence to the coronary arteries during aortic cross-clamping. The composition of the cardioplegic solution varies from centre to centre, but the common constituents are potassium, magnesium and procaine. The solution is infused until the myocardial temperature has dropped to 10°C. Because the aorta is clamped and the solution is aspirated to waste via the coronary sinus, little of it enters the perfusate. Cardioplegic infusion is repeated from time to time to ensure that the myocardial temperature remains below 20°C and that the heart does not commence beating.

Perfusion pressure during bypass is usually kept at 50–70 mmHg. If it rises above this, it may be necessary to add 2.5 mg increments of chlorpromazine to the perfusate, or to infuse sodium nitroprusside. In some centres phentolamine (0.2 mg·kg^{-1}) or phenoxybenzamine (1 mg·kg^{-1}) is added to improve perfusion.

Rewarming is commenced as the intracardiac repair is completed, and this should be performed gradually, with a gradient of not more than 10°C between the temperature of the water in the heat exchanger and the blood. The skin is also rewarmed using the water-blanket. Oesophageal temperature rises faster than nasopharyngeal temperature, and bypass should not be discontinued until the latter has reached 37°C and there is good peripheral circulation. Blood gases and serum potassium level should be checked immediately before coming off bypass, and left atrial (or right atrial after right heart surgery) pressure should be raised to a satisfactory level. This is usually around 10 mmHg for patients with transposition of the great arteries (TGA) but may be as high as 15 mmHg in neonates with total anomalous pulmonary venous drainage. The left atrial pressure line is inserted by the surgeon before bypass is discontinued.

The postperfusion period.   It is wise to ventilate the lungs with 100 per cent oxygen until the haemodynamic state is stable and a satisfactory arterial oxygen tension has been obtained, after which a 50 per cent nitrous oxide/oxygen mixture can be recommenced. Colloidal fluid should be infused to keep the left atrial pressure at a satisfactory level. If the haematocrit is below 40 per cent this fluid should be blood, which should be filtered and warmed. If the haematocrit is above 40 per cent, freshly thawed plasma is preferable. If urine output is below 1 ml·kg⁻¹, either mannitol (0.5 g·kg⁻¹) or frusemide (1 mg·kg⁻¹) may be required. Potassium supplements are required less frequently than for adults. Should blood pressure be low despite adequate filling pressure, it may be necessary to commence inotropic support with dopamine, isoprenaline or, occasionally, adrenaline. These pressor agents should be added to 100 ml of 5 per cent dextrose in a microdrip apparatus (dopamine 6 mg·kg⁻¹ in 100 ml, isoprenaline or adrenaline 0.5–1 mg in 100 ml) and the rate adjusted according to response. (Each microdrop per minute = 1 μg·kg⁻¹ per minute.) If severe hypotension occurs, or if cerebral oedema is anticipated, methylprednisolone sodium succinate may be given in a dose of 30 mg·kg⁻¹.

Heparin reversal is achieved in the usual way with protamine using one and a half to two times the total dose of heparin. Adequacy of neutralization can be confirmed by the ACT.

'Closed heart' procedures

The main 'closed heart' operations performed in the neonatal period are left-to-right shunts, closure of patent ductus arteriosus (PDA) and resection of coarctation of the aorta. The Blalock–Hanlon procedure to increase interatrial mixing of blood has largely been replaced by the balloon atrial septostomy, but is still performed occasionally in some complex congenital heart disease. Shunt operations are still required in a number of neonates.

The increasing use of open heart surgery has made banding of the pulmonary artery to reduce pulmonary blood flow a rarely performed operation.

Pulmonary systemic shunts

The Blalock–Taussig (subclavian to pulmonary artery) shunt is performed on the opposite side to the aortic arch. Occasionally the shunt is established using synthetic material (Gortex). The Waterston (ascending aorta to pulmonary artery) shunt is carried out through a right thoracotomy. Though these shunts are seldom required for tetralogy of Fallot in the neonatal period, they may be used in conditions such as pulmonary atresia with intact ventricular septum.

Cyanosis and polycythaemia are common preoperatively. Hypoxia may be temporarily increased during surgery because of partial occlusion of the pulmonary artery. It is wise to ventilate with 100 per cent oxygen during this period, though this will probably do little to relieve the systemic desaturation. Blood loss should be replaced with plasma because of the high haematocrit. Intra-arterial blood pressure monitoring is not essential, as circulatory collapse is rare. A blood pressure cuff should be placed on the arm opposite to the operative side if a Blalock–Taussig shunt is to be created, as the pulses will be lost on the operative side. Blood pressure should not be allowed to fall below 80 mmHg because of the risk that the shunt may clot. Heparin (1 mg·kg^{-1}) may be required.

Postoperative pulmonary oedema may develop if the shunt is too large. This is more common after a Waterston shunt. Other shunts such as Potts and Glenn shunts are virtually never used nowadays.

Closure of patent ductus arteriosus (PDA)

In approximately 20 per cent of cases a PDA causes persistent chest infection and cardiac failure due to significant left-to-right shunting. These infants are high-risk cases despite preoperative digoxin, diuretics and antibiotics. The operation is performed through a left thoracotomy and no particular problems should be encountered apart from those of the sick neonate in general. Postoperative respiratory failure is common, however, and IPPV may be required for some days.

The presence of a patent ductus arteriosus may be life-saving in neonates who have a severe obstructive lesion in the pulmonary circulation, as in pulmonary stenosis or atresia. Perfusion of the lungs in these cases depends on blood passing from right to left via an atrial or ventricular septal defect, and then via the ductus arteriosus to the pulmonary artery. The closure of the ductus will cause severe hypoxaemia and precipitate the need for surgical intervention. A recent advance has been the ability to keep the ductus open with an intravenous infusion of prostaglandin E in this situation, but it should only be done as a temporary measure while preparations are being made for urgent shunt operation. Occasionally the ductus arteriosus provides the main communication between the pulmonary and systemic circulations in transposition of the great arteries, but oxygenation is achieved more satisfactorily in this condition by mixing pulmonary and systemic blood at atrial level. Balloon atrial septostomy should be performed as soon as possible in all cases of TGA. In coarctation of the aorta the ductus may be carrying much of the blood supply to the lower part of the body. In total anomalous pulmonary venous drainage, the presence of a patent ductus may act as a vent for the congested pulmonary vascular bed. In both these cases, however, urgent surgical correction of the cardiac anomaly is required.

Ligation of the PDA is sometimes required in premature babies with severe hyaline membrane disease. Pulmonary vascular resistance may fall from its initial high level, causing left-to-right shunting through the duct and cardiac failure. If the duct is not ligated at this stage, it may be difficult to wean the baby from controlled to spontaneous ventilation and eventually pulmonary vascular disease will develop.

Coarctation of the aorta

The infantile type of coarctation is commonly preductal, with much of the blood supply to the lower part of the body coming through the patent ductus. Cyanosis is common, due to the high incidence of pulmonary oedema in this condition, and in the worst cases there may be associated hypoplasia of the aortic arch or left ventricle. Other anomalies, such as PDA or ventricular septal defect, may be present. Respiratory and cardiac failure may ensue, with hypoxia and acidosis. Halothane should be avoided as it is very poorly tolerated. The operation is performed through a left thoracotomy, and controlled ventilation with pancuronium is the technique of choice, with 50 per cent nitrous oxide/oxygen if tolerated, though even this sometimes causes hypotension, when 100 per cent oxygen should be used. Intra-arterial pressure monitoring is mandatory, and resuscitation drugs should be immediately available. Acidosis should be corrected before the clamps are applied, and 10–20 ml of blood should be given before they are removed, as even minor degrees of hypovolaemia may cause hypotension. It may be necessary for the surgeons to reclamp the aorta several times before the clamp is finally removed. Postoperative respiratory support for at least 48 hours is essential.

Blalock–Hanlon procedure

This operation was designed to improve interatrial mixing of blood in TGA by the creation of an atrial septal defect. In neonates it is now performed only in cases of complicated TGA. The common method is to expose the right pulmonary artery and veins via a right thoracotomy, and place a clamp on the right and left atrial wall near the interatrial groove so as to include part of the septum in the clamp. The atrium is opened and a portion of septum excised. The clamp is then partially opened, allowing the septum to slip out of it, then quickly reapplied. The snares previously applied to the pulmonary vessels are then released and the atrial incision closed. Alternatively, the operation can be performed after inflow occlusion. Whichever technique is used, it is wise to ventilate the lungs with 100 per cent oxygen for 3 minutes before the clamps are applied, and during closure of the atrium. Major blood loss may occur, and myocardial stimulant drugs should be available. Intra-arterial blood pressure monitoring is mandatory and blood gas and acid–base state should be checked immediately before and after the period of clamping. Controlled ventilation may be required for several days after this procedure.

Pulmonary artery banding

This procedure, which reduces pulmonary blood flow in patients with left-to-right shunts, is nowadays seldom performed in uncomplicated ventricular septal defect (VSD) because the risks of total correction have been reduced to a low level. It is, however, used in complex lesions which are not suitable for early correction, such as a univentricular heart with high pulmonary blood flow, multiple VSD and occasionally VSD with coarctation.

The pulmonary artery is usually approached through a left thoracotomy, though it may be reached from the right. A thick ligature is passed round the artery, and when this is tightened the systemic arterial pressure rises and distal pulmonary artery pressure falls. If the band is applied too tightly, arterial oxygen tension will fall because of inadequate pulmonary blood flow, so intra-arterial pressure monitoring and sampling facilities are mandatory.

Controlled ventilation may be required for several days after this procedure.

Postoperative care

There is a high incidence of postoperative respiratory failure following open heart surgery in the newborn. All neonates are ventilated via a nasotracheal tube for a few hours following open heart surgery, and usually at least until the following morning. The techniques of intubation and ventilation are described elsewhere in this book (p. 157).

Controlled ventilation may also be required after closed heart surgery, particulary banding of the pulmonary artery or the Blalock–Hanlon procedure, where respiratory support may be needed for several days.

During transfer from the operating theatre to the intensive therapy unit the baby should be ventilated with oxygen, and it is wise to monitor precordial heart beat, Doppler blood pressure and ECG. Portable battery-operated machines are now available. Chest drains should be clamped for the shortest possible time, to minimize the risk of tamponade.

In the intensive therapy unit arterial pressure, left atrial and right atrial pressures, heart rate, core and peripheral temperatures should all be monitored continuously after open heart surgery. Urine output and osmolality should be recorded and blood balance charted every 15 minutes. Blood gas and electrolyte measurements should be performed and coagulation status checked. A chest X-ray should be taken as soon as possible to ensure full lung expansion and to check the position of the endotracheal tube in relation to the carina. Blood volume should be maintained according to left atrial pressure and the haematocrit kept between 30 and 40 per cent. Endotracheal suction following the injection of a small volume of saline down the endotracheal tube should be performed every 15 minutes. Careful attention must be paid to the humidification of the inspired gas.

Infants may be sedated with morphine ($0.2 \, mg \cdot kg^{-1}$) or diazepam ($0.2 \, mg \cdot kg^{-1}$) as long as controlled ventilation is being used, but care must be taken with sedation during weaning to spontaneous ventilation. The place of positive end-expiratory pressure (PEEP), intermittent mandatory ventilation (IMV) and continuous positive airway pressure (CPAP) is discussed on p. 160).

Anaesthesia and respiratory obstruction

Table 4.4 Causes of respiratory obstruction

Nasal	May be congenitally absent Choanal atresia
Supraglottic	Pierre Robin syndrome (cleft palate, micrognathia and glossoptosis) Macroglossia—Beckwith syndrome, cretinism Haemangioma Cystic hygroma
Laryngeal	Atresia Laryngomalacia Cleft larynx Laryngeal web Laryngeal oedema Tumours Haemangiomata Associated with raised intracranial pressure, especially in the posterior fossa
Infraglottic	Tracheomalacia, such as at the site of tracheo-oesophageal fistula Tracheal stenosis: congenital or acquired Extrinsic pressure: cyst, tumour, vascular ring

Immediate assessment of severity

Upper airway obstruction, if severe and prolonged, may cause serious hypoxia, which can easily be fatal, or may lead to cerebral ischaemia and resultant mental retardation. The fact that a high proportion of infants with Pierre Robin syndrome are found later to have mental retardation may be due to hypoxia subsequent to severe and prolonged episodes of airway obstruction. The immediate assessment of the severity of the obstruction must be based on a rapid and thorough appraisal of the clinical signs and recent history. The amount of stridor is not on its own the most significant feature, as infants with epiglottitis can be severely ill without much stridor, and infants with acute laryngotracheobronchitis (croup) who are not so ill can have marked inspiratory stridor. Any infant able to take a feed without undue distress is unlikely to require urgent treatment though other signs may show that immediate action is necessary to relieve the obstruction. These signs include severe intercostal and subcostal recession, paradoxical movement of the chest and abdomen, with abdominal protrusion on inspiration, tracheal tug, sweating, cyanosis, peripheral hypoperfusion, head retraction, or difficulty or inability to take a feed. Arterial blood gases tend initially to be well maintained though hypercarbia, hypoxia and metabolic acidosis develop in sequence, as respiratory failure ensues. It is important to remember that the higher alveolar ventilation of the infant—two to three times that of the adult—results in lower ranges of carbon dioxide content in arterial blood and that levels above 5.7 kPa (40 mmHg) are abnormally elevated for an infant. However, such levels are initially well tolerated and an elevated Pa_{CO_2} itself is not necessarily an indication for active intervention.

Cardiovascular deterioration occurs early in severe respiratory obstruction with initial tachycardia, pallor or cyanosis, progressing to bradycardia and cardiac arrest. Cardiac arrest is particularly likely to result in brain damage if it has been preceded by a period of severe hypoxaemia, which is usually the case in respiratory obstruction.

Clinical examination usually gives a clue to the site and possible cause of obstruction. There may be an obvious external abnormality such as malformation of the nares, micrognathia, cleft palate or swellings around the neck and face (Figs. 4.15 and 4.16).

Nasal obstruction by choanal atresia may be fatal, as the neonate is an obligatory nose breather. Extreme respiratory distress with cyanosis is characteristically relieved when the infant cries, thus using its mouth for breathing.

Choanal atresia is ruled out by passing soft rubber catheters through both

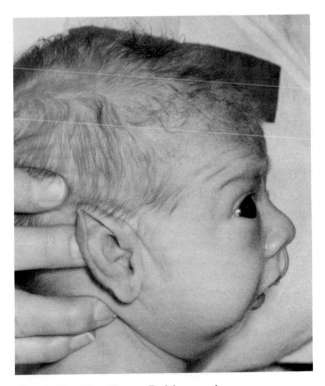

Fig. 4.15 The Pierre Robin syndrome.

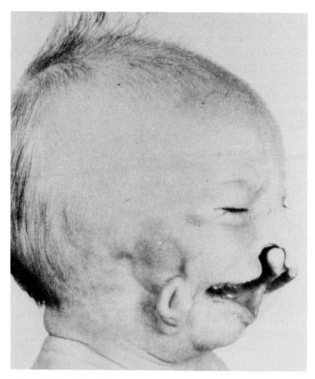

Fig. 4.16 The Treacher-Collins syndrome.

nostrils. In cases of severe airway obstruction the airway may have to be established before accurate diagnosis is made.

Inspiratory stridor is said to be characteristic of pathology of the larynx, which narrows or collapses on inspiration. Both inspiratory and expiratory stridor are heard with obstructive lesions below the larynx.

Diagnostic investigations may include X-rays of the face, neck and chest, and xerography of the upper airway (Fig. 4.17). Barium swallow may show displacement by tumours or abnormal vascular structures. Propyliodone (Dionosil) swallow investigations should be carried out only when a skilled anaesthetist can be standing by with a full resuscitation kit. Laryngoscopy and endotracheal intubation may be necessary in order to suck out any aspirated Dionosil and relieve hypoxia.

Management of respiratory obstruction

Intubation, laryngoscopy, bronchoscopy or tracheostomy may be necessary for the management of these cases. Nasal obstruction may be relieved by the insertion of an oral airway which must be strapped in place, as it will otherwise be rejected by the baby. Babies with gross nasal deformities, though rare, may need an urgent tracheostomy.

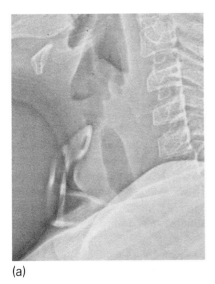
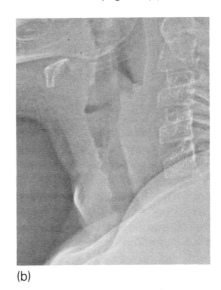

(a)   (b)

Fig. 4.17 Xerograms showing (a) complete respiratory obstruction due to subglottic stenosis, and (b) the same child after relief of the obstruction by laryngotracheoplasty. (Courtesy of J. N. G. Evans)

The obstruction associated with micrognathia (e.g. Pierre Robin syndrome) may be relieved by nursing in the prone position; more rarely, it may need a nasopharyngeal airway or, very rarely indeed, tracheostomy. A nasopharyngeal airway is a satisfactory alternative to suturing the tongue forwards onto the mandible.

Bronchoscopy and laryngoscopy should never be undertaken lightly—especially in the neonate. Bronchoscopy is never indicated merely for removal of secretions. It should never be performed in the presence of tracheal infection or subglottic stenosis, as oedema and stridor will be intensified.

Laryngoscopy

Some of the conditions for which laryngoscopy is performed can progress to partial or complete respiratory obstruction under anaesthesia; this applies particularly to patients with micrognathia, large tongues, rigid jaws, and pharyngeal or glottic cysts or tumours. A selection of laryngoscopes and endotracheal tubes of various lengths must be on hand and a surgeon must be ready to perform a tracheostomy if that becomes urgently necessary. Great care must be taken to maintain the infant's body temperature during the induction and surgery, and ECG and precordial stethoscope should be employed. Premedication consists only of atropine, and this should always be given because local topical analgesia is essential and only works well if adequate drying of secretions has been achieved. In spite of the advantages generally cited for controlled ventilation in neonatal anaesthesia, these are usually outweighed by spontaneous ventilation in anaesthesia for laryngoscopy. Spontaneous ventilation is mandatory in respiratory obstruction unless the anaesthetist is certain he will be able to inflate the lungs of the paralysed patient. In children with laryngeal papillomata or cystic hygroma the movements which occur around the glottis during spontaneous breathing, with possible bubbles of saliva, may provide the only means of identification of the laryngeal inlet.

Laryngoscopy is usually performed with oxygen and halothane anaesthesia via a well fitting face mask. The application of a constant distending pressure by controlling the gas leak from the open-ended T-piece reservoir bag is sometimes extremely useful during induction in cases of respiratory obstruction, and may even lead to the complete disappearance of stridor. It is essential therefore that the mask used is one which can make a good seal with the face: the Rendell–Baker mask is not ideal for this purpose, and one with an inflatable rim is preferable, despite its larger dead space. It may be impracticable to cannulate a vein before induction of anaesthesia but a vein should be cannulated as soon as possible after induction. Topical 4 per cent lignocaine (3–5 mg·kg^{-1}) is sprayed into the larynx and trachea when the patient is fairly deeply anaesthetized, and at this time the anaesthetist can make a first assessment of the larynx. The commonly used proprietary lignocaine (Xylocaine) spray delivers 10 mg aliquots. If microlaryngoscopy is to be performed it is wise to intubate the trachea first, in order to assess the diameter of the larynx and upper trachea, and to provide a secure airway while the microscope is set up. A small nasotracheal tube is convenient for this purpose. This is usually withdrawn into the nasopharynx during the microlaryngoscopy, and oxygen and halothane are insufflated through it. Spontaneous ventilation allows the surgeon to observe the movements of the larynx during the procedure, and this is essential in the diagnosis of prolapsing larynx, laryngomalacia, cleft larynx and vocal cord palsy.

The Sanders injector cannot be used during larygoscopy in infants because it cannot be easily fitted to the microlaryngoscope blade, and there is often difficulty in aiming the jet directly down the larynx. There is also a risk of seeding papillomata further down the airway. Intratracheal jets have been used in older children, but are dangerous if the cords close, and should not be used in neonates.

Controlled ventilation through a small nasotracheal tube will be required for the occasional patient in respiratory failure.

Bronchoscopy

Anaesthetic techniques for bronchoscopy depend on the apparatus available. Paediatric bronchoscope systems such as the Storz (Fig. 4.18) are supposed to be 'ventilating' bronchoscopes, but it is very unwise to give relaxants to the patient during such an endoscopy unless one is sure that it is possible to inflate the lungs adequately through the bronchoscope. Assisted or spontaneous ventilation is possible using an anaesthetic T-piece on the side arm of the infant bronchoscope. The smaller sized bronchoscopes have very little gap within the bronchoscope when the telescope is in place and no ventilation is possible in these circumstances. Manual ventilation is not possible during suction and insertion of the telescopes, during which time a paralysed patient would become increasingly hypoxic. Bronchoscopy is performed under general anaesthesia with full local anaesthesia to the respiratory tract as described above, and oxygen and halothane delivered to the side arm of the bronchoscope, ventilation being spontaneous or gently controlled.

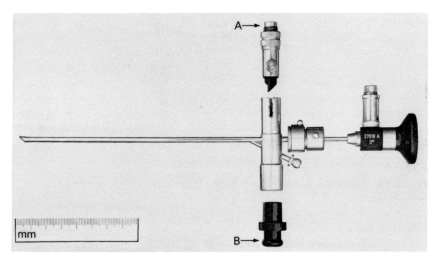

Fig. 4.18   The Storz bronchoscope, showing (A) light carrier and (B) the attachment for anaesthetic T-piece.

Monitoring must include ECG and precordial stethoscope; if a hand is placed over the epigastrium, each breath can be felt and the thumb on the apex can feel each heart beat. It is useful to attach two precordial stethoscopes—one on the left for breath and heart sounds, and the right only for breath sounds. This allows monitoring of respiration to both lungs and is especially useful when the bronchoscope is down one or other main bronchus.

The Sanders jet, which uses the Venturi principle, is seldom used for infant bronchoscopy because most endoscopists prefer the superior optical characteristics of modern fibreoptic telescopic bronchoscopes. These bronchoscopes are expensive, however, and not available in all centres. Bronchoscopy for inhaled foreign body, for example, may require the use of the Negus bronchoscope (Fig. 4.19), and when this is used, ventilation with the Venturi is preferable to spontaneous breathing. Ideally, the anaesthetic technique should allow the surgeon to change from one type of bronchoscope to another. Chest wall movements should be carefully monitored whichever technique is used. Pneumothorax is a theoretical complication of the Venturi jet, but hypoxia from inadequate ventilation is probably a more likely hazard.

Standard pipeline pressures may be used safely if the Venturi needle in infants does not exceed 19 s.w.g. Anaesthesia can be maintained if the entrained gas includes oxygen and halothane to the side arm of the Negus-type bronchoscope.

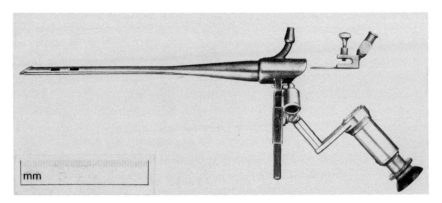

Fig. 4.19 The Negus suckling bronchoscope with Venturi attachment.

Pneumothorax is a complication of bronchoscopy whichever anaesthetic technique is used. Blood gas analysis has shown that ventilation with a Sanders type of Venturi is satisfactory unless the patient has severe chronic respiratory disease with markedly reduced lung compliance.

Most laryngotracheal lesions are diagnosed by laryngoscopy or bronchoscopy. The characteristic small, floppy glottis and epiglottis of laryngomalacia and vocal cord palsies will be observed. Tracheomalacia is seen during spontaneous ventilation and extrinsic compressions may be present. Pulsatile swellings may be vascular in origin, though such pulsation may be transmitted and is not therefore diagnostic of a vascular origin. If the compression is caused by an aberrant subclavian artery causing a vascular ring, the pressure of the tip of the bronchoscope may cause changes in the character of the radial pulses. This condition usually requires a cine swallow with contrast medium, using the image intensifier to visualize the obstruction and so make for a definitive diagnosis.

After the examination, the patient should be placed in the lateral position, the lower side being the side of any bleeding from trauma or biopsies. The patient must be observed until he is *fully* awake as stridor and respiratory distress may not reappear until then.

Bronchoscopy may precipitate complete respiratory obstruction in very marginal cases by minimal oedema caused by the instrumentation. Bronchoscopy is not necessary and may be dangerous in the diagnosis of subglottic stenosis. Postoperatively the baby is nursed in a head box with humidified air or air and oxygen mixture, and should have nothing by mouth until 3 hours after the lignocaine spray to the glottis. Dexamethasone should be given (p. 195) for laryngeal oedema if stridor reappears.

Vascular ring

A vascular ring is most commonly due to persistent right and left aortic arches, but can also be caused by a right sided aortic arch and left patent ductus arteriosus or ligamentum arteriosum, or by aberrant right subclavian, innominate or left common carotid arteries. The trachea and oesophagus are enclosed within the vascular ring, and pressure on the trachea causes the main clinical problem, airway obstruction. This usually develops within the first few weeks after birth, is exaccerbated by feeding, and may become very severe. The clinical picture is that of intrathoracic respiratory obstruction, with a croaking cry, brassy cough, signs of hyperinflation of the chest, expiratory wheezes and rhonchi. Respiratory infections are common, and the diagnosis should be considered in cases of repeated chest infection. In severe cases the infant may adopt the hyperextended posture of opisthotonus, and sudden death from respiratory obstruction may occur. Associated cardiac anomalies may be present, particularly ventricular septal defect or bicuspid aortic valve.

Diagnosis should be confirmed as soon as possible, either by endoscopy or cine swallow, and treatment is surgical. Since the airway obstruction is low in the trachea it may occasionally be necessary to use a long endotracheal tube passed into the right main bronchus, with a side hole cut 1.5 to 2 cm from the tip to allow ventilation of the left lung. Care should be taken not to pass too large a tube through the obstructed area because of the risk of oedema causing postoperative stridor, and it is better to keep the tube above the lesion if possible. Surgical manipulation may cause complete airway obstruction, and severe haemorrhage may occur.

Symptoms of airway obstruction may be slow to improve postoperatively, as the trachea has often been severely distorted and some degree of tracheomalacia is almost always present. The infant should be nursed in a humidified head box with some oxygen enrichment, and may be helped by dexamethasone (0.25–0.5 mg·kg^{-1}). In severe cases, continuous positive airway pressure, either using nasal prongs or a small endotracheal tube may be necessary. Tracheostomy may have to be considered, though the low position of the obstruction often makes this unsatisfactory. The possibility of incomplete resection of vascular ring should be considered if postoperative respiratory obstruction persists, as in some cases a ligamentum arteriosum may be responsible for continuing symptoms.

Choanal atresia

If this condition is complete, obstruction by bony or membranous walls will cause severe respiratory distress in the newborn. An oral airway is inserted and fastened by tapes to the baby's cheeks until he comes to the anaesthetic room. Transnasal or transpalatal puncture and dilatation is usually performed at the age of 1–2 days.

Premedication is with atropine, and intubation is performed awake after preoxygenation through the oral airway. A 3 mm (internal diameter) Oxford tube is used and a small throat pack inserted. The T-piece will come down over the patient's chest. Ventilation is controlled using a relaxant technique with all the precautions necessary for neonatal anaesthesia and surgery. After the nasal punctures are completed, the surgeon inserts short plastic tubes which remain in place in the nose for 6 weeks. The operation usually takes 20–30 minutes. The patient is extubated fully awake after removal of the throat pack and careful suctioning of the pharynx. Pulmonary aspiration of regurgitated stomach contents is very likely to occur after this operation and careful nursing observation must start at once in the postoperative ward.

Tracheostomy

This is very rarely an emergency procedure. With the advent of long-term nasotracheal intubation, tracheostomy is never required nowadays merely for respiratory support in the neonatal period. The indications for tracheostomy vary from centre to centre, but it is generally accepted that for ventilator-dependent patients tracheostomy may be delayed for many weeks and then performed, not for airway reasons but because handling, nursing and stimulating a growing baby are easier with a tracheostomy. Tracheostomy is most commonly performed for conditions of the upper airway for which endotracheal intubation is unsuitable, such as subglottic stenosis, severe tracheomalacia or vocal cord palsy.

Many patients who require tracheostomy already have an endotracheal tube in place. Premedication is with atropine, and preoxygenation is followed by intubation if a tube is not already in place. A very small tube may be necessary in cases of subglottic stenosis. A relaxant technique with controlled ventilation may be used. The patient is positioned with a sandbag behind the neck to extend the head maximally and to throw the trachea into prominence. Monitoring must include ECG and oesophageal stethoscope. Infant tracheostomy is a very specialized and difficult operation. Cartilage must never be excised because of the risk of subsequent tracheal collapse and stenosis, nor must the incision be too high in the trachea because of the risk of subglottic stenosis. The surgeon usually makes a vertical incision through the second and third tracheal rings. If it is made lower than this, there is a risk of endobronchial intubation or tube dislodgement. Some surgeons insert two 'stay sutures' which remain in place for 7 days until the tube is changed for the first time. The patient is ventilated with 100 per cent oxygen before the tracheal incision is made and the tube withdrawn only enough for the tracheostomy tube to be inserted. The uncuffed tracheostomy tube is chosen, usually one size larger than the endotracheal tube in place, and then a check is made that all connections are available and that they fit. The Great Ormond Street (Aberdeen) non-cuffed plastic tracheostomy tube (3.5–7 mm plain) is very satisfactory, though at the moment no

British Standard connections are available for them (Fig. 4.20). Anaesthesia is continued through the tracheostomy with a sterile connector. The tube must fit with a comfortable air leak around it and be fixed tightly round the neck with tapes.

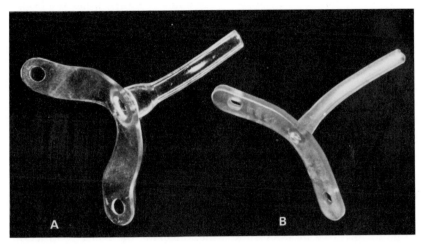

Fig. 4.20 Neonatal tracheostomy tubes: A, Great Ormond Street pattern; B, Portex.

Postoperatively a chest X-ray is taken to check the position of the tip of the tube.

The complications of tracheostomy are more severe than those of endotracheal intubation. Accidental dislodgement in the first week before a track is established can be disastrous, though less so if stay sutures are employed. Severe infection, tracheal granuloma and vascular erosion are reported complications.

A tracheostomy mask with humidified air is used to prevent crusting of secretions in the tube. Eventually the epithelium in the trachea becomes stratified and humidification is usually discontinued after about 3 weeks.

References and further reading

Surgical emergencies

Arthur, D. S. (1980). Caudal anaesthesia in neonates and infants. *Anaesthesia* (in press).

Collins, D. L., Pomerance, J. J., Travis, K. W., Turner, S. W. and Papperbaum, S. J. (1977). A new approach to congenital posterolateral diaphragmatic hernia. *Journal of Pediatric Surgery* **12**, 149.

Cullum, A. R., English, I. C. W. and Branthwaite, M. A. (1973). Endobronchial intubation in infancy. *Anaesthesia* **28**, 66.

Dibbins, A. W. (1976). Neonatal diaphragmatic hernia: a physiological challenge. *American Journal of Surgery* **131**, 408.

Girven, D. P., Webster, D. M. and Shandling, B. (1974). The treatment of omphalocele and gastroschisis. *Surgery, Gynecology and Obstetrics* **139**, 222.

Inkster, J. (1976). Paediatric anaesthesia and intensive care. In: *Recent Advances in Anaesthesia and Analgesia, 12.* Ed. by C. Langton Hewer and R. S. Atkinson. Churchill Livingstone, Edinburgh and London.

de Lorimer, A. A., Tierney, D. F. and Parker, H. R. (1967). Hypoplastic lungs in fetal lambs with surgically produced congenital diaphragmatic hernia. *Surgery* **62**, 12.

Martin, J. T. (1976. Case history number 93: congenital lobar emphysema. *Anesthesia and Analgesia* **55**, 869.

Nixon, H. H. (1978). *Surgical Conditions in Paediatrics.* Butterworths, London.

Rickham, P. P., Lister, J. and Irving, I. M. (Eds) (1978). *Neonatal Surgery*, 2nd edn. Butterworths, London.

Salem, M. R., Wong, A. Y., Lin, Y. H., Firor, H. V. and Bennett, E. J. (1973). Prevention of gastric distension during anesthesia for newborns with tracheo-esophageal fistula. *Anesthesiology* **38**, 82.

Sears, B. E., Carlin, J. and Tunell, W. P. (1978). Severe congenital subglottic stenosis in association with congenital duodenal obstruction. *Anesthesiology* **49**, 214.

Thomas, D. F. M. and Atwell, J. (1976). The embryology and surgical management of gastroschisis. *British Journal of Surgery* **63**, 893.

Waterston, D. J., Bonham Carter, R. E. and Aberdeen, E. (1962). Oesophageal atresia: tracheo-oesophageal fistula: a study of survival in 218 infants. *Lancet* **i**, 819.

Anaesthesia for neuroradiology and neurosurgery

Creighton, R. E., Relton, J. E. S. and Meridy, H. W. (1974). Anesthesia for occipital encephalocoele. *Canadian Anaesthetists' Society Journal* **21**, 403.

Fitch, W. and McDowall, D. G. (1971). Anaesthesia for neuroradiological investigations. *Proceedings of the Royal Society of Medicine* **64**, 75.

Lassen, N. A. and Christensen, M. S. (1976). Physiology of cerebral blood flow. *British Journal of Anaesthesia* **48**, 719.

Leading article (1977). Screening for neural tube defects. *Lancet* **i**, 1345.

Michenfelder, J. D., Gronert, G. A. and Rehder, K. (1969). Neuro-anesthesia. *Anesthesiology* **30**, 65.

Anaesthesia for cardiac surgery

Abbott, T. R. (1977). Oxygen uptake following deep hypothermia. *Anaesthesia* **32**, 524.

Bailey, L. L., Takeuchi, Y., Williams, W. G., Trusler, G. A. and Mustard, W. T. (1976). Surgical management of congenital cardiovascular anomalies with the use of profound hypothermia and circulatory arrest. Analysis of 180 consecutive cases. *Journal of Thoracic and Cardiovascular Surgery* **71**, 485.

Barratt-Boyes, B. G., Simpson, M. and Neutze, J. M. (1971). Intracardiac surgery in neonates and infants using deep hypothermia with surface cooling and limited cardiopulmonary bypass. *Circulation* **43**, 44.

Battersby, E. F., Hatch, D. J. and Towey, R. M. (1977). The effects of prolonged nasotracheal intubation in children. A study in infants and young children after cardiopulmonary bypass. *Anaesthesia* **32**, 154.

Cooper, D. K. C. (1979). Study of the factors contributing to the mortality associated with open heart surgery in infants. *Thorax* **34**, 138.

Ebert, P. A. (1978). Aspects of myocardial protection. *Annals of Thoracic Surgery* **26**, 495.

Elliott, R. B., Starling, M. B. and Neutze, J. M. (1975). Medical manipulation of the ductus arteriosus. *Lancet* **i**, 140.

English, I. C. W., Frew, R. M., Piggott, J. F. and Zaki, M. (1964). Percutaneous catheterisation of the internal jugular vein. *Anaesthesia* **24**, 521.

Glover, W. J. (1977). Management of cardiac surgery in the neonate. *British Journal of Anaesthesia* **49**, 59.

Hatch, D. J., Cogswell, J. J., Taylor, B. W., Battersby, E. F., Glover, W. J. and Kerr, A. A. (1973). Continuous positive airway pressure after open heart operations in infancy. *Lancet* **ii**, 469.

Johnston, A. E., Radde, I. C., Steward, D. J. and Taylor, J. (1974). Acid–base and electrolyte changes in infants undergoing profound hypothermia for surgical correction of congenital heart defects. *Canadian Anaesthetists' Society Journal* **21**, 23.

Keith, J. D., Rowe, R. D. and Vlad, P. (Eds) (1978). *Heart Disease in Infancy and Childhood*, 3rd edn. Macmillan, New York.

Kirklin, J. W. (1973). *Advances in Cardiovascular Surgery*. Grune & Stratton, New York.

Leading article (1975). Congenital heart disease: Incidence and aetiology. *Lancet* **ii**, 692.

Lippmann, M., Nelson, R. J., Emmanouilides, G. C., Diskin, J. and Thiebault, D. W. (1976). Ligation of patent ductus arteriosus in premature infants. *British Journal of Anaesthesia* **48**, 365.

Pang, L. M. and Mellins, R. B. (1975). Neonatal cardiorespiratory physiology. *Anesthesiology* **43**, 171.

Pick, M. J., Hatch, D. J. and Kerr, A. A. (1976). The effects of positive end expiratory pressure on lung mechanics and arterial oxygenation after open heart surgery in young children. *British Journal of Anaesthesia* **48**, 983.

Stark, J. (1980). Current status of cardiac surgery in early infancy. *Proceedings of the 8th European Congress of Cardiology*, Paris, 22nd–26th June 1980, p. 253. Karger, Basel.

Stranger, P., Heymann, M. A., Tarnoff, H., Hoffmann, J. I. E. and Rudolph, A. M. (1974). Complications of cardiac catheterization of neonates, infants and children—a three-year study. *Circulation* **50**, 595.

Subramanian, S., Wagner, H., Vlad, P. and Lambert, E. (1971). Surface-induced deep hypothermia in cardiac surgery. *Journal of Pediatric Surgery* **6,** 612.

Wakusawa, R., Shibata, S. and Okada, K. (1977). Simple deep hypothermia for open heart surgery in infancy. *Canadian Anaesthetists' Society Journal* **24,** 491.

Anaesthesia for bronchoscopy

Miyasaka, K., Sloan, I. A. and Froese, A. B. (1980). Evaluation of jet injector Sanders' technique for bronchoscopy in paediatric patients. *Canadian Anaesthetist's Society Journal* **27,** 117.

5

Postoperative care

Introduction

Neonatal intensive care, where the neonatal paediatrician, anaesthetist and surgeon must work together as part of a multidisciplinary team, is a large and expanding subject which we have not attempted to cover in this book. We have, however, tried to bring together in this chapter those aspects of basic postoperative care which we feel are essential to the safe practice of neonatal anaesthesia, many of which have been touched on in previous chapters.

Postoperative respiratory failure

Aetiology

Respiratory failure may occur as a result of medical, surgical, neurological, metabolic or renal disease, and supportive therapy must be accompanied by the appropriate treatment of the underlying disease.

The neonate has limited reserves of lung function. Oxygen consumption per unit of body weight is approximately twice that of the adult, and any increase may lead to inadequate tissue oxygenation. The increase in oxygen consumption which occurs in response to cold has been described on p. 19, and the importance of taking every precaution to avoid heat loss from a neonate has been stressed. The baby should be covered with warm Gamgee or similar material as soon as the operation has finished, and returned to an incubator or placed under a heat canopy as soon as possible. Even inside an incubator the temperature can be hostile to the naked neonate, especially if premature.

Severe hypoxaemia may result from increase in the work of breathing, reduction in ventilation/perfusion ratio in the lungs, pulmonary venous congestion or oedema, or from intrapulmonary or intracardiac right-to-left shunting. Failure of oxygen transport may also cause tissue hypoxia, as in hypovolaemia, cardiac failure, hypotension, red cell haemolysis or reduced 2,3-DPG content of blood. Hypoxaemia may occur secondary to hypoventilation in cases of postanaesthetic depression, intracranial haemorrhage, raised intracranial pressure or neurological degenerative conditions such as Werdnig–Hoffmann's disease.

Intrapulmonary shunting may occur when the already small functional residual capacity (FRC) is reduced. This is more likely to happen after intrathoracic operations or after major intra-abdominal surgery where the diaphragm may be forced upwards by pressure from below. Severe disturbances in lung function may follow cardiac surgery in the newborn because of reduced compliance and lung volume and increased resistance, with consequent increase in the work of breathing. In other babies, pre-existing respiratory problems—such as surfactant deficiency causing alveolar instability in hyaline membrane disease (HMD), pulmonary hypoplasia in cases of congenital diaphragmatic hernia, meconium aspiration or lung soiling in oesophageal atresia—may be the main factor contributing to postoperative respiratory failure.

Assessment

It is clear that the above factors contribute to postoperative respiratory therapy being required relatively frequently in the neonate. In a recent series of admissions to the neonatal surgical intensive care unit at Great Ormond Street, 21.2 per cent of babies required intermittent positive pressure ventilation (IPPV) after non-cardiac surgical operations (Table 5.1).

Table 5.1   Admissions to a neonatal surgical unit 1974–1977 (excluding myelomeningocele)

Diagnosis	No.	Ventilated	Deaths
Abdominal surgery:			
General	165	15 (9.1%)	14 (8.5%)
Exomphalos	22	2 (9.1%)	2 (9.1%)
Gastroschisis	15	9 (60.0%)	5 (33.3%)
Tracheo-oesophageal fistula/atresia	69	17 (24.6%)	9 (13.0%)
Diaphragmatic hernia	36	21 (58.6%)	13 (36.1%)
Miscellaneous	18	5 (27.8%)	4 (22.2%)
Total	325	69 (21.2%)	47 (14.5%)

The criteria for IPPV after neonatal surgery vary from centre to centre. Most people agree that a period of IPPV is desirable after open heart surgery in neonates, and almost always after closed heart surgery because, if this is required in the first month of life, it suggests that the baby is extremely sick. Opinions vary widely, however, about the place of IPPV after non-cardiac surgery in the neonate. A few advocate elective ventilation after almost all operations whilst others confine this approach to high-risk groups of neonates such as those with congenital diaphragmatic hernia, oesophageal atresia or gastroschisis. Yet others decide each case on clinical grounds, and this has been the approach generally adopted by the present authors in recent years, with results which compare favourably with those published by others.

Though a well conducted general anaesthetic should have little effect in itself on postoperative lung function in the neonate, each case must be carefully assessed at the end of surgery. A decision not to ventilate post-operatively should be postponed until it is clear that adequate spontaneous ventilation has returned, and that the baby stays well oxygenated when breathing room air. If there is any doubt about the adequacy of respiration–whether because of hypothermia, residual narcosis, incomplete reversal of muscle relaxants or any other factor—postoperative IPPV should be used.

Clinical and radiological assessment

Whatever ventilatory policy is adopted, clinical assessment supported by blood gas and acid–base analysis is central to good respiratory care. Even in babies ventilated electively, weaning from IPPV must be controlled clinically. Signs of respiratory failure must be accurately assessed after weaning in case a return to IPPV is indicated. Increasing respiratory frequency and pulse rate are early clinical signs of respiratory difficulty, often accompanied by some evidence of increase in the work of breathing, such as flaring of the alae nasi, grunting and intercostal recession. A respiratory frequency above 60 breaths per minute suggests fairly severe respiratory distress. The degree of spontaneous activity, including crying and ability to accept a feed, should be carefully recorded, and responsiveness to simple manoeuvres such as the taking of blood pressure should be noted. Restlessness should be regarded as a sign of hypoxia unless proved otherwise. Periodic respiration is not uncommon in the newborn, especially if premature, and has been discussed on p. 11. Apnoeic spells lasting longer than 10 seconds, sometimes accompanied by bradycardia or cyanosis, are probably pathological, so increasing duration or frequency of attacks may be an indication for IPPV. Because of the close relationship between respiratory and cardiovascular failure, respiratory assessment must always include observation of pulse rate. The state of the peripheral circulation is assessed by the quality of the peripheral pulses and temperature of the skin.

Repeated clinical assessment, preferably by the same person, is essential in deciding whether a baby is improving or deteriorating; babies should not be allowed to accumulate secretions or to become exhausted. Any sudden deterioration should raise the possibility of pneumothorax or hypoglycaemia. A chest X-ray may exclude or confirm the presence of cardiomegaly, collapsed areas of lung, pneumothorax or collection of fluid. Elevation of one side of the diaphragm after thoracic surgery suggests the possibility of phrenic nerve damage.

Blood gas analysis

Arterial blood gas and acid–base estimations provide essential support to, but do not replace, clinical judgement. Babies who, after surgery, are not maintaining an arterial oxygen tension between 6.7 and 10.7 kPa (50–80 mmHg) when breathing oxygen-enriched mixtures or whose arterial carbon dioxide tension is rising above 6.7 kPa (50 mmHg) are likely to require ventilatory assistance, though sometimes IPPV is indicated on purely clinical grounds, even in the presence of relatively normal blood gases.

In the newborn, repeated arterial blood samples may be obtained by catheterization of an umbilical artery. An electrode is available which can be inserted into the artery to provide continuous measurement of oxygen and carbon dioxide tensions if required. The umbilical and lower limb arteries will contain a lower arterial oxygen tension than upper limb arteries if there is significant right-to-left shunting through a patent ductus arteriosus. Femoral artery puncture carries the risk of prejudicing the blood flow to the limb and also the possibility of causing a septic arthritis in the hip. If repeated samples are required later in the neonatal period, it may be necessary to insert a small cannula (22 s.w.g.) into the radial artery. This can usually be done percutaneously. The oxygen tension samples taken during crying is of little value and it is always wise to record the inspired oxygen concentration at the time of sampling.

The measurement of cutaneous oxygen and carbon dioxide tensions has recently become practicable due to improvements in the design of heated skin electrodes and advances in mass spectrometry. A reasonable correlation has been found between cutaneous and arterial gas levels when the peripheral circulation is good, though this may not be maintained when peripheral circulation fails, during periods of hypotension or in patients with generalized cutaneous dilatation as occurs with tolazoline therapy. The effect of nitrous oxide can be minimized by keeping the polarizing voltage below 600 mV.

Whilst clinical assessment of respiratory failure, supported by radiological and blood gas data, is essential, there are occasions—particularly in chronic pulmonary disease and in the management of infants on IPPV—when a more objective assessment of resistance, compliance and lung volume is useful. For this reason, methods of measurement of these parameters are described briefly below.

Lung mechanics

Resistance.   Airways resistance alone may be measured with a whole body plethysmograph. In this technique, which has now been modified for babies, the subject breathes quietly from a heated circuit containing a pneumotachograph whilst enclosed in an air-tight chamber. Airways resistance is calculated from the simultaneous measurement of flow from the pneumotachograph and of pressure changes within the chamber. The inspired gas must be heated to 37°C and humidified to prevent these pressure changes being affected by differences between inspired and expired gas volumes. Measurement of the resistance of the airways plus lung tissue, known as *total pulmonary resistance*, may be obtained using the simultaneous measurement of flow and oesophageal pressure (Fig. 5.1). The former signal can be obtained from a pneumotachograph and the latter from a thin-walled oesophageal balloon (Fig. 5.2).

Oesophageal balloons for use in the newborn must be carefully made, and each one's static and dynamic accuracy should be checked. The volume of

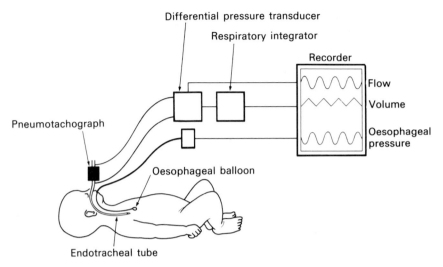

Fig. 5.1 System for assessing respiratory function in babies.
(From Hatch, 1975)

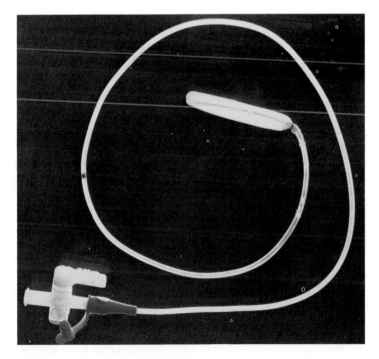

Fig. 5.2 Oesophageal balloon.

air to be used in a balloon should be determined from the *in vitro* pressure/ volume curve; the best results are obtained with balloons of 30–50 mm length, and with a diameter of 7.5 mm and a wall thickness of 0.045–0.075 mm mounted on a 5 FG catheter and connected to a suitable pressure transducer. The balloon should be inserted into the lower oesophagus and its position checked by ensuring that mouth pressure changes and oesophageal pressure changes recorded simultaneously are identical when the subject attempts to breathe against an occluded airway. Resistance is usually measured at the mid-point of inspiration and expiration.

Compliance.   Compliance, or lung stiffness, is measured by volume change per unit pressure change. An estimation of compliance may be obtained using the pneumotachograph and oesophageal balloon system described above if the basic assumption is made that there is no air flow at end-tidal points (Fig. 5.3). Dynamic compliance measurements obtained in this way will be erroneous when resistance is high or during rapid rates of breathing, and in these circumstances static measurements give more reliable information about the elastic properties of the lungs. The classic method of measuring static compliance by inflating the lungs with known volumes of air from a calibrated syringe is of limited clinical use because it requires general anaesthesia, muscle relaxation and a non-leaking airway. The use of a

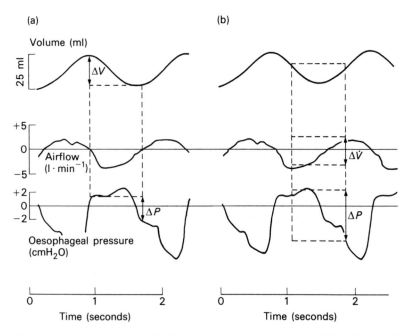

Fig. 5.3   Calculation of (a) dynamic compliance, $\Delta V/\Delta P$, at points of zero flow, and (b) total pulmonary resistance, $\Delta P/\Delta V$, at points of mid volume.

respiratory jacket to measure thoracic volume change overcomes these difficulties. The thin-walled rubber jacket covers the chest and abdomen and is inflated to $3\,cmH_2O$. During quiet breathing, small pressure changes occur in the jacket and these can be calibrated by the injection of known volumes of air from a side arm syringe. Static compliance is measured by recording changes in thoracic volume when stepwise changes in pressure are applied to the airway. These pressure changes can be applied in apnoeic patients by holding the reservoir bag of a T-piece circuit at a constant pressure for 2 or 3 seconds at the end of each inflation and then allowing the pressure to drop to atmospheric (Fig. 5.4). In spontaneously breathing patients the stepwise pressure change can be produced from a large pressurized reservoir drum. The technique can be used via an endotracheal tube or using a face mask.

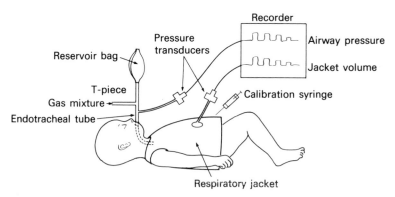

Fig. 5.4 Measurement of static compliance using the respiratory jacket. (Courtesy of B. W. Taylor)

Lung volumes. Since compliance and resistance (or, more commonly, its reciprocal conductance) are volume-dependent it is helpful to know the lung volume at which these measurements are made. Values of compliance divided by lung volume are referred to as 'specific compliance'. Lung volume measurements are also valuable in their own right because abnormalities, either reductions or increases, may be of clinical significance. There are two main techniques for the measurement of lung volume.

1. *Dilution techniques.* These rely on the dilution of known quantities of an inert gas with the air contained in the lungs. They do not measure any air in the chest which is not in communication with the major air passages. The volume obtained by these measurements is known as the functional residual capacity (FRC). The principal techniques used are the closed circuit helium method and the open circuit nitrogen washout method, both of which have been adapted for use in young children.

2. *Whole body plethysmography* (Fig. 5.5).   Lung volume is calculated from changes in pressure recorded simultaneously at the mouth and within the plethysmograph when the subject attempts to breathe against a temporary obstruction. This technique measures all gas within the chest at the time of measurement including any contained in lung cysts or other areas of lungs which are not in communication with the major air passages. The measurement obtained is usually referred to as thoracic gas volume (TGV).

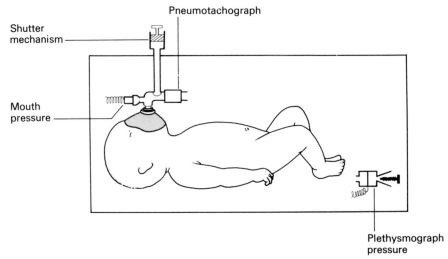

Fig. 5.5   Infant whole body plethysmography.

Management

Oxygen therapy

An increased inspired oxygen concentration is essential for many babies postoperatively—after thoracotomy or major abdominal surgery, after large blood transfusions or if respiratory distress is present. A head box is necessary to achieve steady concentrations over 60 per cent. The gases should be fully humidified to about 34°C using a heated water-bath type of humidifier at a flow of 6 litres per minute to prevent accumulation of carbon dioxide. If cold oxygen is used, there will be stimulation of the trigeminal area of the face and an undesirable increase in metabolic oxygen demand. Both inspired oxygen concentration and the resultant Pao_2 must be closely monitored (p. 81). High inspired oxygen concentrations are implicated in the production of lung damage. Bronchopulmonary dysplasia is probably caused by several factors such as high ventilatory pressures, high inspired oxygen concentrations, chronic infection and poor mucociliary function. Prolonged alveolar concentrations in excess of 60 per cent oxygen are implicated, though the relative importance of each of the factors is not known. High inspired oxygen concentrations are used as necessary to give as normal a Pao_2 as possible, though not if the low Pao_2 is caused by a fixed intracardiac right-to-left shunt as in transposition of the great arteries (TGA).

Infants of less than 36 weeks' gestational age are at risk from cicatricial retrolental fibroplasia caused by vasoconstrictive effects in the retinal vessels of high Pao_2. The safe level of Pao_2 and duration of effect are unknown but it is wisest to aim for a Pao_2 of 9.3–10.7 kPa (70–80 mmHg). Other factors such as blood flow, temperature, haematocrit and metabolic activity must operate because the condition is reported in patients who have never received an increased inspired oxygen concentration and also in patients with cyanotic congenital heart disease.

Nasotracheal intubation

If the infant is to be intubated postoperatively for IPPV or constant distending pressure (see below), it is usual to change the tube from an orotracheal to a nasotracheal for what may be prolonged respiratory support. The nasal route is generally preferred because of the superior fixation, greater comfort and ease of nursing, including improved mouth care.

With the oral endotracheal tube still in place and an assistant ventilating the baby, an uncut 3 mm (or 2.5 mm) plain PVC (tissue tested) nasotracheal tube is lubricated and passed through the nares as far as the glottis. This is done using a laryngoscope. The endotracheal tube is cut to the desired length so that its tip lies mid-way between the glottis and the carina—an extra 2 cm on the length of the tube. A Tunstall connection (Figs. 5.6 and 5.7) is fixed into the tube and, as the oral tube is removed by the assistant, the nasal tube is inserted through the glottis using intubating forceps and

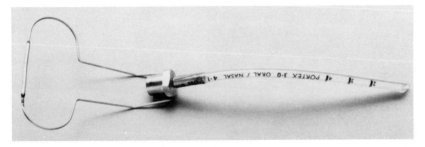

Fig. 5.6 Plain Portex tube with Tunstall connector.

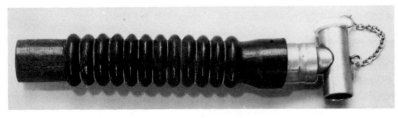

Fig. 5.7 Catheter mount with Oxford swivel connector.

then secured as shown in Fig. 5.8. Auscultation should reveal bilateral air entry and a check chest X-ray should show the tip of the endotracheal tube lying in the mid-point of the trachea. The correct size of endotracheal tube is that which allows normal controlled ventilation with the application of constant distending pressure if this is required, but which allows a slight air leak at an airway pressure of 25–30 cmH$_2$O. The leak must be present at all times and checked daily. If the leak disappears (subglottic oedema), this is an indication for the endotracheal tube to be changed to one a size smaller (not smaller than 2.5 mm internal diameter). It is our practice to change the tube from one nostril to the other every 10 days to preserve the symmetry of the nostrils. After this length of time, the plastic of the tube hardens as plasticizers are leached out.

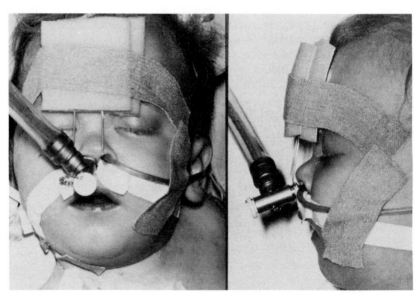

Fig. 5.8 Fixation of the Tunstall connector. (From Hatch, 1977)

With meticulous care it is possible to use endotracheal tubes for respiratory support for very prolonged periods, with a very low complication rate. Tracheostomy is usually preferred when an artificial airway is required for more than a few weeks, as it is more convenient for the nurses and enables the patient to become more mobile.

All the complications of endotracheal intubation are avoidable.

1. *Dislodgement* by accident is prevented by firm fixation of the tube. Such an accident need not be a disaster in a good intensive care unit, especially when the use of muscle relaxants is restricted to those patients who cannot be adequately ventilated without them.

2. *Blockage* of the tube by inspissated secretions is avoided by humidifica-

tion of the inspired gases to full saturation at a temperature approaching that of the body (35–44 mg of water vapour per litre gas flow at 37°C = 80–100 per cent relative humidity). Most commercial humidifiers do not come up to these standards, and some of the water vapour condenses in the patient tubing. We thus find it necessary to instill 0.5 ml physiological saline down the endotracheal tube every 30 minutes, followed by suction using a sterile soft rubber catheter. Suctioning is potentially hazardous, as it may introduce infection; disposable gloves should be worn and a sterile technique used. It may cause dangerous hypoxia because ventilation is discontinued and intrapulmonary oxygen concentration is reduced; suction time should be limited to 15 seconds. Techniques do exist whereby suctioning can take place while IPPV continues and negative pressure is minimized in the airways if the diameter of the suction catheter does not exceed 70 per cent of the endotracheal tube diameter—this is difficult when small endotracheal tubes are used. Suction can also cause traumatic lesions of the tracheal mucosa, but these are minimized if soft rubber catheters with an end hole (not whistle-tip) are used.

The nursing staff should always know the exact length of the endotracheal tube and ensure that the suction catheter passed is longer than this, otherwise secretions at the tracheal end of the tube may not be reached.

3. *Subglottic stenosis* is potentially the most serious complication, resulting from the use of a tube which is too tight in the cricoid ring. Pressure on the mucosa causes necrosis and, later, fibrosis. This is entirely avoidable if a tube is used with a small air leak around it and the air leak is maintained at all times. In our series of 3000 babies and children with prolonged intubation over the past 6 years there has been no case of subglottic stenosis.

4. *Postextubation stridor* occurs rarely and is most commonly seen after short intubations (24–36 hours). Very rarely does the condition require reintubation, but usually responds to dexamethasone 0.25 mg·kg^{-1} intravenously, followed by 0.1 mg·kg^{-1} 6-hourly intramuscularly for 12 hours.

5. *Nasal ulcers*. There is a small incidence of nasal ulcers even with careful technique. These heal normally if the tube is changed to the other nostril.

Intubated patients should also receive chest physiotherapy as a prophylactic measure, and all the techniques of physiotherapy—vibration, percussion, manual lung expansion—are applicable to the neonate, though care must be taken. There is no place for bronchoscopy for removal of secretions or for treatment of lobar consolidation. These conditions are more safely dealt with by intubation and physiotherapy.

Because of the *very* low morbidity of endotracheal intubation in all sizes of neonates it is our practice to institute mechanical ventilation or constant distending pressure (CDP) only after the patient has been intubated. This is not necessarily the practice in other centres where babies are ventilated (at low pressures only) with face masks and CDP is applied through nasal prongs. Securing the airway by endotracheal intubation has the additional advantage of allowing full tracheal toilet.

Mechanical ventilation

Most mechanical ventilators which can deliver a low flow rate are suitable for paediatric use and success often depends more on the skill and judgement of the medical and nursing staff than on the characteristics of a particular machine. Major criteria for the choice of ventilator must include reliability, an efficient humidifier, accurate control of inspired oxygen concentration, a reliable alarm system and ease of sterilization between cases. Suitable machines include Siemens' Servo 900B (Fig. 5.9) and Bourn's BP200 (Fig. 5.10), the latter having many very important characteristics for mechanical ventilation of the neonate. Formulae or nomograms to work out ventilator settings are unhelpful, as they seldom take account of either the compressed gas effect of the machine, the humidifier and the patient tubing, or the very reduced lung compliance of many of the patients, both of which need extra volume not calculated in a nomogram. A tidal volume of $10 \, ml \cdot kg^{-1}$ and a respiratory rate of 30 breaths per minute are suitable initial

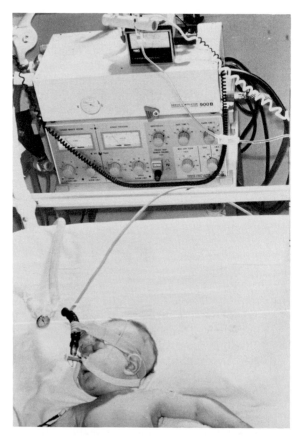

Fig. 5.9 The Servo Ventilator 900B (Siemens).

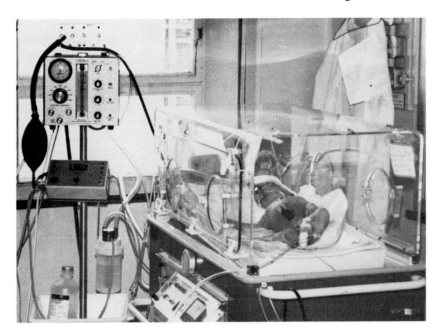

Fig. 5.10 The Bourn Ventilator BP200.

settings (or, alternatively, a peak inflating pressure of 20–25 cmH$_2$O), but it is essential to check the adequacy of chest movement at once. Initially, a clinical assessment of ventilatory adequacy is made, but it is confirmed by blood gas analysis later. Blood gas measurements are used for monitoring ventilatory progress. Most babies are easily managed with small doses of morphine (0.2 mg·kg^{-1} i.m. or i.v.) or diazepam (0.2 mg·kg^{-1} i.m. or i.v.). If mechanical ventilation is instituted for postoperative respiratory failure, the relaxants used intraoperatively are not reversed. However, it is otherwise rarely necessary to paralyse babies for mechanical ventilation. Pancuronium 0.1 mg·kg^{-1} is needed in certain circumstances where a harmful drive to ventilation cannot easily be obtunded. It may be required in severe states of respiratory and metabolic acidosis, with low cardiac output, persistent hypoxia causing restlessness or in situations where patients are being deliberately hypoventilated to prevent lung damage from excessive ventilatory pressures.

When ventilating newborn babies, it is essential to minimize the possibility of lung damage known as bronchopulmonary dysplasia (BPD) or ventilator lung (Fig. 5.11). Factors associated with the production of this fibrosis and cyst formation, with destruction of the lung architecture and hence its function, are high ventilatory pressures, high inspired oxygen concentrations, poor mucociliary function and chronic infection. The condition is often progressive, as increasing ventilation/perfusion mismatching requires increasing inspired oxygen concentrations and falling lung compliance

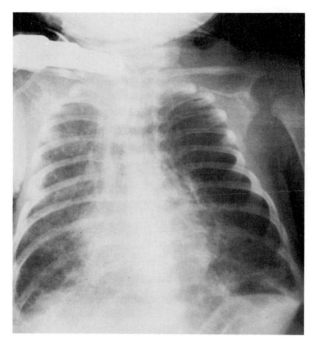

Fig. 5.11 Bronchopulmonary dysplasia. X-ray showing grossly overinflated lungs and evidence of severe parenchymal damage.

needs higher inflation pressures. Because of the great capacity of the infant lung to regenerate, the condition need not be fatal, if factors known to cause BPD are minimized. Recovery will be slow.

Modern neonatal ventilators have a variety of facilities which help to minimize bronchopulmonary dysplasia, as discussed below.

The ventilatory *rate* is usually set at 30, which is less than the respiratory rate of spontaneous breathing. It is generally agreed that alveolar ventilation is better at lower frequencies. The rate must be related to the inspiratory/expiratory time ratio; otherwise, insufficient time is available for expiration if the respiratory rate is too high. The machine must have the facility for rates up to 60 per minute because increasing the rate from 30 is a way of reducing the peak inflation pressure in babies with low pulmonary compliance.

The method of cycling the machine is relevant, because pressure generators produce a square wave of pressure which is advantageous in ventilating the very stiff lungs of babies with hyaline membrane disease, so that the alveoli are kept distended during inspiration and gas exchange is improved.

Flexible inspiratory/expiratory times ratios are important because a reversal of I/E ratio from 1:2 to 2:1 may help to improve gas exchange in patients with hyaline membrane disease (though not necessarily in patients with other lung pathology) (Table 5.2). Very little of the mean increased

Table 5.2 The effect of reversal of the I/E ratio on oxygenation

	Hyaline membrane disease (age 1 day)		Bronchopulmonary dysplasia (age 4 months)	
Time	15.00	16.00	11.45	12.57
I/E	1 : 2	2 : 1	1 : 2	2 : 1
Fio_2	1.0	1.0	0.55	0.55
Frequency	36	36	30	30
pH	7.05	7.25	7.33	7.27
$Paco_2$	9.3 kPa (70 mmHg)	5.1 kPa (38 mmHg)	5.9 kPa (44 mmHg)	6.5 kPa (49 mmHg)
Base excess	−15.9	−12	−3.5	−6.3
Pao_2	2.0 kPa (15 mmHg)	8.0 kPa (60 mmHg)	14 kPa (105 mmHg)	7.2 kPa (54 mmHg)

intrapulmonary pressure is transferred to the mediastinum, when the lungs are stiff, so little effect on the cardiac output is to be expected. As the lungs improve, the mean intrathoracic pressure must be reduced. Alterations in I/E ratio may allow the inspired oxygen concentration to be reduced to potentially less toxic levels.

Positive end-expiratory pressure (PEEP).   A ventilator must have the facility for application of PEEP (this is the accepted term for constant distending pressure applied during controlled ventilation). The ability of a constant distending pressure to improve arterial oxygenation at a given inspired oxygen concentration depends on the relationship between functional residual capacity (FRC) and the closing volume (CV) in the lungs. When closing volume exceeds FRC, airway closure occurs during tidal breathing (as in young children). This increases both right-to-left intrapulmonary shunting and the alveolar–arterial oxygen gradient (A–aDo$_2$). The effect is greater in pathological states of the lung associated with fluid retention. With the application of a constant distending pressure, alveoli in the mid-region of the lungs open (those in the dependent parts of the lungs are already maximally taking part in ventilation), thus increasing FRC in relation CV, decreasing intrapulmonary shunting and decreasing A–aDo$_2$ (so-called alveolar recruitment). Early application of constant distending pressure to neonatal lungs affected by hyaline membrane disease improves the gas exchange and may decrease the severity of the disease by reducing surfactant consumption. The net effect of PEEP on oxygen delivery to the tissues is variable and depends on a balance of factors, including possible reduction of the cardiac output in hypovolaemic patients or after cardiac surgery. Levels of PEEP up to 8–10cmH$_2$O are used in an attempt to lower the required inspired oxygen concentration. Higher levels of PEEP increase the risk of alveolar rupture and tension pneumothorax.

Maintenance ventilation should aim for as low a peak inflation pressure as possible, preferably less than 30cmH$_2$O, and as low an inspired oxygen concentration as possible using the techniques described to provide a Pao_2 of

8–10.7 kPa (60–80 mmHg). The continuing need for high airways pressure and a high Fio_2 are discouraging signs.

Weaning.   Some programme for discontinuing mechanical ventilation in stages is started when cardiovascular, biochemical and neurological stability is achieved and when $Paco_2$ is less than 6.7 kPa (50 mmHg) and Pao_2 more than 10.7 kPa (80 mmHg) at an Fio_2 of 0.5 with peak inflation pressures less than 25 cmH$_2$O.

Weaning may be a protracted affair if the lungs are infected, if there is significant cardiac failure or if bronchopulmonary dysplasia ensues. A tracheostomy may eventually be necessary (p. 144). Because of the great potential for regeneration of the infant lung, with patience it is often possible to wean from the ventilator even the most difficult case.

It is important not to leave babies breathing through an endotracheal tube without end-expiratory pressure, particularly those with low pulmonary compliance. Zero end-expiratory pressure allows the stiff lungs to collapse progressively so that closing volume encroaches further on the functional residual capacity with increasing right-to-left intrapulmonary shunting and hypoxaemia. As lung volume falls, airways resistance to gas flow rises, increasing the work of breathing and the oxygen consumption. This will increase any hypoxia already present. With an endotracheal tube in place, the normal glottic mechanism whereby an infant can generate 2–3 cmH$_2$O end-expiratory pressure is lost. The grunting, so characteristic of infants with respiratory distress, is thought to be an attempt to overcome the cause of the distress by delaying alveolar emptying and minimizing the time during which airway closure can occur.

Constant positive airway pressure (CPAP; constant distending pressure during spontaneous ventilation).   This is now always used for weaning small patients from ventilators and also for respiratory support in some patients who do not need mechanical ventilation. CPAP may be delivered via nasotracheal tube, nasal prongs, face mask or a head box with a tight seal around the neck. All methods have advantages and disadvantages, so the choice depends on the practice in a particular centre. CPAP is successful in improving Pao_2 in infants with right-to-left intrapulmonary shunts through areas of atelectasis which are perfused but not oxygenated. Additionally, CPAP, because it keeps small airways distended, causes a fall in pulmonary resistance which in turn reduces the work of breathing and thus the oxygen consumption. Recurrent apnoea is not a contraindication to the use of CPAP because apnoea may be improved by activation of sensory stretch receptors. The ventilation is shifted to a higher point in the pressure/volume curve, thus increasing functional residual capacity and oxygenation.

CPAP can be applied using either a modified T-piece circuit as in (Fig. 5.12) or a modified Bain circuit which relies on a fresh gas flow of three times the patient's minute volume. On the expiratory side, a water manometer is used to read the pressure and is a safety 'blow off' valve to avoid excessive pressures within the circuit. A reservoir bag with a controlled leak acts to

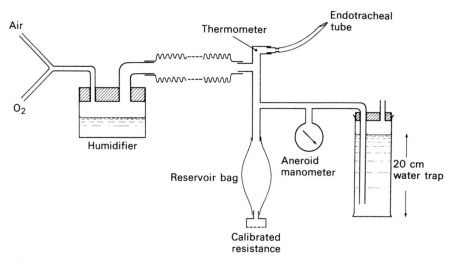

Fig. 5.12 Modified T-piece circuit used for application of CPAP. (From Hatch *et al.*, 1973)

smooth the level of pressure and prevents gross fluctuations within the circuit.

A distending pressure of 6–8 cmH$_2$O pressure is suitable to begin with, though this is gradually reduced in a stepwise fashion after the inspired oxygen concentration has been reduced to 40 per cent or lower. Patients are extubated from levels of 2 cmH$_2$O CPAP. The incidence of pneumothorax with CPAP is estimated to be as high as 6 per cent, and suitable equipment for relief of pneumothorax must be at hand. Transillumination of the thorax using a fibrelight lead is a useful technique for immediate diagnosis of a pneumothorax. In an emergency, a short needle should be inserted into the pleural cavity through the second intercostal space in the mid clavicular line and the air aspirated. A formal chest drain should then be inserted and connected to an underwater seal. During the weaning process careful monitoring must be made of the clinical and blood gas state of the patient. Particularly important are the rate of respiration and the assessment of the work of breathing.

Intermittent mandatory ventilation (IMV). Neonatal ventilators should now be fitted with integral CPAP mechanisms to facilitate the weaning process, and indeed most use IMV. This mode involves mandatory lung inflations provided by the ventilator at preset tidal volumes in between which the patient breathes spontaneously at constant distending pressure. As the patient improves, it is possible to decrease gradually the number of mandatory breaths until ventilatory support is completely withdrawn. The patient is then breathing from a CPAP circuit. Systems which rely on a continuous fresh gas flow (e.g. Bourn's) are better than those in which the flow is of a demand type (e.g. Servo).

Extubation is carried out when the patient has been breathing spontaneously for several hours at a CPAP of 2 cmH$_2$O and has a satisfactory Paco$_2$ with an inspired oxygen concentration of less than 40 per cent. After extubation there may be temporary incompetence of the larynx and impaired ciliary function. Pulmonary atelectasis is very common and repeated intubation may be required for physiotherapy and suction. Occasionally, temporary support with CPAP via nasal prongs is needed until the competence of the glottis is restored. Bronchoscopy is never necessary merely to remove secretions or to expand collapsed lobes.

Intravenous feeding

Fluid balance and intravenous feeding

The principles of intravenous therapy are discussed on p. 52, but a general guide for postoperative fluid management is to give approximately 3 ml·kg^{-1} per hour intravenously for the period in which no oral intake is possible. A suitable solution for maintenance therapy is 4 per cent dextrose with 0.18 per cent saline, though abnormal losses such as gastric aspirate should be replaced with physiological saline and potassium and calcium supplements administered as indicated by the serum electrolyte values.

Such a regimen is inadequate in its calorific value and will not sustain growth so is used only for short periods of time. In some infants after major surgery or with necrotizing enterocolitis, protracted diarrhoea, extreme prematurity or renal failure parenteral nutrition is required, sometimes for very prolonged periods.

Maintenance of complete intravenous feeding requires the strictest of aseptic techniques and intensive nursing care. Frequent biochemical monitoring is necessary using microtechniques which allow tests to be performed on very small volumes of blood. Acidosis and dehydration must be corrected before commencing intravenous feeding, especially when hypertonic or fructose-containing solutions are used. Fat emulsions are contraindicated in patients with hyperlipidaemia and in the presence of poor bone marrow function. They may be used cautiously in patients with mild liver dysfunction, though daily estimations of liver transaminases should be made. Infused fat should be rapidly cleared from the circulation. If the serum becomes turbid, this suggests that too much fat is being given.

Solutions are pumped at a constant rate into the superior vena cava or right atrium through a long Silastic catheter, using pumps such as the Ivac. To minimize the risk of infection, the catheter is tunnelled subcutaneously for some distance before it enters the vein and a bacterial filter is fitted into the system as near the patient as possible. (Intralipid will not pass through bacterial filters.) The catheters are usually inserted surgically, though it is possible to pass a catheter through a 19 s.w.g. scalp vein needle in a scalp or arm vein, when it can be expected to pass centrally on a flow-guided principle. Some centres recommend that peripheral veins should be used on a rotational basis and that the site of venepuncture be changed every 24 hours. The inclusion of Intralipid in doses of 4 g fat·kg^{-1} body weight each day (non-irritant to veins) has meant that peripheral veins may be used for longer periods before resorting to central veins where risks of infection and serious venous thrombosis are greater.

Regimens are available which are effective in maintaining positive nitrogen balance and growth for many months. The caloric requirement is not less than $420\,MJ\cdot kg^{-1}$ ($100\,kcal\cdot kg^{-1}$) body weight per 24 hours.

Solutions for complete intravenous feeding include:

1. *Amino acid solutions*, of which several are commercially available. All solutions also contain a non-nitrogenous source of calories such as glucose, ethanol or sorbitol. The L-forms of the amino acids are more effective in maintaining positive nitrogen balance (e.g. Vamin). In addition to the eight amino acids essential for adult growth, histidine, proline, alanine and cystine are essential for infant growth. Aminosol–fructose–ethanol (AFE) and Vamin contain all the amino acids for the growing infant, but the osmolality of these two solutions is very high. They are, however, the most appropriate solutions for use in infancy, but their infusion rate should not exceed AFE $48\,ml\cdot kg^{-1}$ and Vamin $72\,ml\cdot kg^{-1}$ per day, as the fructose they contain will cause metabolic acidosis. In practice, Vamin with Glucose is the most satisfactory solution for use in infants.

Table 5.3 The constituents of Vamin with Glucose

Presentation

Clear, straw-coloured solutions for intravenous use containing pure crystalline L-amino acids together with glucose and added electrolytes to the following formula:

L-Alanine	3.0 g	L-Proline	8.1 g
L-Arginine	3.3 g	L-Serine	7.5 g
L-Aspartic acid	4.1 g	L-Threonine	3.0 g
L-Cysteine/Cystine	1.4 g	L-Tryptophan	1.0 g
L-Glutamic acid	9.0 g	L-Tyrosine	0.5 g
Glycine	2.1 g	L-Valine	4.3 g
L-Histidine	2.4 g	Glucose	100.0 g
L-Isoleucine	3.9 g	Sodium	50 mmol
L-Leucine	5.3 g	Potassium	20 mmol
L-Lysine	3.9 g	Calcium	2.5 mmol
L-Methionine	1.9 g	Magnesium	1.5 mmol
L-Phenylalanine	5.5 g	Chloride	55 mmol

in each 1000 ml (pH 5.2). Sterile and pyrogen-free.

Nitrogen per litre: 9.4 g, corresponding to about 60 g of first-class protein.
Caloric content per litre: 650 Kcal., of which 410 Kcal. are provided by glucose.

(Courtesy of Kabi Vitrum Ltd.)

2. *Fat emulsions*. Intralipid is the usual fat solution used (as 10 or 20 per cent), prepared from fractionated soybean oil and in the form of triglycerides. The fat is rapidly cleared from the plasma, even in the newborn, at a rate of up to $8\,g\,fat\cdot kg^{-1}$ body weight per 24 hours. The addition of heparin

may increase the clearance rate of the fat but this is controversial. The infusion of fat is restricted to 4 g fat·kg⁻¹ per day at a rate not exceeding 0.5 g fat·kg⁻¹ per hour. The solution is usually introduced at 1 g·kg⁻¹ per day, and if the serum is not turbid then the amount is increased.

3. *Monosaccharides*. There is no agreement as to which source of calories is preferable. Fructose is said to be less irritant to veins and is less dependent on insulin for its further metabolism. Urinary losses of fructose are greater than glucose and the former may therefore result in a greater osmotic diuresis. Hypoglycaemia may occur during fructose infusion, so at least 50 per cent of the infused carbohydrate should be given as dextrose.

Ethyl alcohol is included in AFE as 2.5 g·dl⁻¹. Its toxicity is a limiting factor in infancy and its inhibitory action on antidiuretic hormone causes increased urinary losses of water and electrolytes.

Vitamins are required, though exact requirements are not well worked out. A multivitamin infusion is given in a dose of 3 ml per day with folic acid 0.5 mg per day, vitamin K 3 mg twice weekly and vitamin B_{12} 100 µg once monthly. If intravenous feeding is continued for more than 1 week, biotin 0.5 mg per day and choline chloride 150 mg per day must be given.

Weekly infusions of plasma 10 ml·kg⁻¹ will provide the necessary trace metals (Table 5.4).

The volumes of each nutrient are increased daily, with maximum volumes being achieved on the fourth day. On the first day, one-third of the total requirements (150 ml·kg⁻¹ per 24 hours) are given as 20 per cent Intralipid, 15 per cent glucose, and Vamin with Glucose, the remaining fluid being given as 4 per cent dextrose with 0.18 per cent saline. On the second day, the volumes are doubled and if the clinical and biochemical state of the patient is satisfactory, then full volumes are achieved after 4 days (Fig. 5.13).

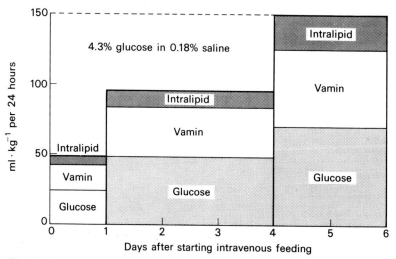

Fig. 5.13 A technique for the introduction of infusates for complete intravenous feeding in infants. (From Harries, 1971)

Table 5.4 A regimen for complete intravenous feeding of infants (all values per kg per 24 hours)

Solution	Volume (ml)	Calories	Amino acids (g)	Na$^+$ (mmol)	K$^+$ (mmol)	Cl$^-$ (mmol)	Ca^{2+} (mmol)	Mg^{2+} (mmol)
Vamin	50	34	3.5†	2.5	1.0	2.5	0.125	0.075
15% Glucose	70	42						
20% Intralipid	20	36						
MgSO$_4$ (0.5 mmol Mg^{2+}·ml^{-1})	0.3							0.150
K$_2$HPO$_4$ (1 mmol K$^+$·ml^{-1})	1.0				1.0			
10% Calcium gluconate (0.25 mmol Ca^{2+}·ml^{-1})	3.5						0.875	
Total	145.3*	102	3.5	2.5	2.0	2.5	1.0	0.225

* Due to osmotic diuresis total fluid volume may need to be increased using 4% dextrose in 0.18% saline.
† Caloric value included in total calories.

(From Harries, 1971)

Small volumes of each solution are given in a rotational system so that an even distribution of solutions during a 24-hour period is achieved. For example:

Vamin with Glucose	30 ml	for	1 hour
Dextrose 15%	30 ml		1 hour
Intralipid	10 ml		$\frac{1}{2}$ hour
0.18% Saline	30 ml		1 hour
Vamin with Glucose	30 ml		1 hour etc.

A series of three-way stopcocks is arranged to which the required number of drip sets can be attached.

No solutions, drugs or electrolytes may be added to Intralipid or to amino acid or carbohydrate infusions. Vitamins and electrolytes are given into the infusion chamber containing dextrose–saline, but each electrolyte solution must be given separately or precipitation may occur with mixtures. The daily requirements of Ca^{2+} and K^+ must be given in spaced doses to obviate the danger of cardiac arrhythmia with excessive concentrations.

All infusion tubing, drip sets and solutions are changed every 24 hours. If possible, limited oral feeding should be continued during total intravenous feeding, even with severe diarrhoea, to maintain a continuous 'trophic' stimulus to the small intestinal mucosa. Intraluminal substrates exert a trophic effect on the small intestinal mucosa, the effect being mediated by gastrointestinal hormones such as gastrin.

Intravenous alimentation must not be withdrawn abruptly or hypoglycaemia may develop. High levels of circulating insulin are stimulated by the infusions and the levels persist after withdrawal of the feeding. Oral feeding should be reintroduced over several days before the intravenous alimentation is withdrawn.

Complications of intravenous alimentation are very common and include septicaemia with organisms such as *Candida albicans*, *Staphylococcus aureus* and *Escherichia coli*. All procedures are undertaken with the strictest of aseptic precautions. Topical antibiotics combined with nystatin at the point of skin entry may reduce the incidence of infections. Central venous catheters must be removed if blood cultures are found to be positive. Small neonates are especially vulnerable to infections, and it has also been postulated that metabolic changes accompanying the correction of malnutrition may predispose the infant to infection. Marked electrolyte disturbances and severe acidosis are sometimes seen. Phlebitis and venous obstruction are common, though the incidence is reduced by including isotonic fat emulsions in the regimen (e.g. Intralipid). Catheter dislodgement may occur, with extravasation of solutions into the surrounding tissues.

As most of the amino acid solutions contain relatively high sodium concentrations and are markedly hyperosmolar, excess may cause oedema and cardiac failure.

Intravenous feeding can be expected to provide all the nutrient agents essential for normal growth in the small baby, including the essential amino acids and agents required for brain cell replication and maturation of the central nervous system. Levels of amino acids which are too low or too high may produce irreversible brain damage in young infants. High circulating levels of blood ammonia have been reported in infants given intravenous feeding and this, too, is a potential source of brain injury.

References and further reading

Respiratory failure—assessment

Auld, P. A. M., Nelson, N. M., Cherry, R. B., Rudolph, A. J. and Smith, C. A. (1963). Measurement of thoracic gas volume in the newborn infant. *Journal of Clinical Investigation* **42**, 476.

Beardsmore, C. S., Helms, P., Stocks, J., Hatch, D. J. and Silverman, M. (1980). Improved esophageal balloon technique for use in infants. *Journal of Applied Physiology* (in press).

Chiswick, M. L. and Milner, R. D. G. (1976). Crying vital capacity. Measurement of neonatal lung function. *Archives of Disease in Childhood* **51**, 22.

Conway, M., Durbin, G. M., Ingram, D., McIntosh, N., Parker, D., Reynolds, E. O. R. and Soutter, L. P. (1976). Continuous monitoring of arterial oxygen tension using a catheter tip polarographic electrode in infants. *Pediatrics* **57**, 244.

Cook, C. D., Sutherland, J. M., Segal, S., Cherry, R. B., Mead, J., McIlroy, M. B. and Smith, C. A. (1957). Studies of respiratory physiology in the newborn infant. III. Measurements of mechanics of respiration. *Journal of Clinical Investigation* **36**, 440.

Eberhard, P. and Mindt, W. (1978). Reliability of cutaneous oxygen measurement by skin sensors with large-size cathodes. *Acta Anaesthesiologica Scandinavica* (Suppl.) **68**, 20.

Fox, W. W., Schwart, J. G. and Shaffer, T. H. (1977). A new approach for measuring functional residual capacity (FRC) in the intubated infant. *Pediatric Research* **11**, 570.

Gerhardt, T., Bancalari, E., Cohen, H. and Maciar-Loza, M. (1977). Respiratory depression at birth—value of Apgar score and ventilatory measurements in its detection. *Journal of Pediatrics* **90**, 971.

Hatch, D. J. (1975). The measurement of pulmonary function. In: *Recent Advances in Paediatric Surgery, 3*. Ed. by A. W. Wilkinson. Churchill Livingstone, Edinburgh and London.

Hatch, D. J. and Taylor, B. W. (1976). Thoracic gas volume in early childhood. *Archives of Disease in Childhood* **51**, 859.

Huch, A. and Huch, R. (1977). Technical, physiological and clinical aspects of transcutaneous Po_2 measurements. In: *Non-invasive Clinical Measurement*. Ed. by D. E. M. Taylor and J. Whamond. Pitman Medical, Tunbridge Wells.

LeSoeuef, P. N., Morgan, A. K., Soutter, L. P., Reynolds, E. O. R. and Parker, D. (1978). Comparison of transcutaneous oxygen tension with arterial oxygen tension in newborn infants with severe respiratory illnesses. *Pediatrics* **62**, 692.

Milner, A. D., Hull, D., Hatch, D. J. and Cogswell, J. J. (1972). A new method for measuring static compliance in infants and young children. *Clinical Science* **43,** 689.

Peabody, J. L., Willis, M. M., Gregory, G. A., Tooley, W. H. and Lucey, J. F. (1978). Limitations and advantages of transcutaneous oxygen electrodes. *Acta Anaesthesiologica Scandinavica* (Suppl.) **68,** 76.

Phelan, P. D. and Williams, H. E. (1969). Ventilatory studies in healthy infants. *Pediatric Research* **3,** 425.

Respiratory failure—management

Aberdeen, E. (1965). Tracheostomy care in infants. *Proceedings of Royal Society of Medicine* **58,** 900.

Battersby, E. F., Hatch, D. J. and Towey, R. M. (1977). The effects of prolonged naso-endotracheal intubation in children: a study in infants and young children after cardio-pulmonary bypass. *Anaesthesia* **32,** 154.

Downes, J. J. (1974). Intermittent mandatory ventilation. *Archives of Surgery* **109,** 519.

Downes, J. J. and Raphaely, R. C. (1975). Pediatric intensive care. *Anesthesiology* **43,** 238.

Gregory, G. A., Kitterman, J. A., Phibbs, R. H., Tooley, W. H. and Hamilton, W. K. (1971). Treatment of idiopathic respiratory distress syndrome with continuous positive airways pressure. *New England Journal of Medicine* **284,** 1333.

Hatch, D. J. (1977). Anaesthesia for cardiac surgery in the first year of life. In: *Anaesthesia for Cardiac Surgery and Allied Procedures.* Ed. by M. A. Branthwaite. Blackwell Scientific, Oxford.

Hatch, D. J., Cogswell, J. J., Taylor, B. W., Battersby, E. F., Glover, W. J. and Kerr, A. A. (1973). Continuous positive airway pressure (CPAP) after open heart operations in infancy. *Lancet* **ii,** 469.

Hayes, B. and Robinson, J. S. (1970). The assessment of methods of humidification of inspired air. *British Journal of Anaesthesia* **42,** 94.

James, L. S. and Lanman, J. T. (Eds) (1976). Symposium: Retrolental fibroplasia. *Pediatrics* **57,** Supplement, 591.

Mackersie, A. M., Hatch, D. J. and Farnsworth, G. M. (1980). Ventilatory management of neonates undergoing surgery. *British Journal of Anaesthesia* **52,** 273.

Phibbs, R. H. (1977). Oxygen therapy: a continuing hazard to the premature infant. *Anesthesiology* **47,** 486.

Reynolds, E. O. R. and Taghizadeh, A. (1974). Improved prognosis of infants mechanically ventilated for hyaline membrane disease. *Archives Disease in Childhood* **49,** 505.

Roberton, N. R. C. (1976). CPAP or not CPAP? *Archives of Disease in Childhood* **51,** 161.

Stocks, J. G. (1972). The management of respiratory failure in infancy. *Anaesthesia and Intensive Care* **1,** 486.

Sumner, E. and Frank, J. D. (1980). The effect of tolazoline on the treatment of congenital diaphragmatic hernias. A report of its successful use to reverse a transitional circulation in four patients. *Archives of Disease in Childhood* (in press).

Workshop on Bronchopulmonary Dysplasia (1979). *Journal of Pediatrics* **95,** 815.

Intravenous feeding

Baum, J. D. and Aynsley-Green, A. (1975). Intravenous feeding in children. *Clinical Trials Journal*, Suppl. 1, **114.**

Harries, J. T. (1971). Intravenous feeding in infants. *Archives of Disease in Childhood* **46,** 855.

Harries, J. T. (1978). Aspects of intravenous feeding in childhood. In: *Advances in Parenteral Nutrition*. Ed. by Ivan Johnston. MTP Press, Lancaster.

Pildes, R. S., Cornblath, M., Warren, I., Page-El, E., di Menza, S., Morrit, D. M. and Peeva, A. (1974). A prospective controlled study of neonatal hypoglycemia. *Pediatrics* **54,** 5.

6

Resuscitation of the newborn

Asphyxia at birth

Approximately 5 per cent of newborn infants fail to breathe immediately after delivery, and more than 50 per cent of the deaths in the first week of life occur in this group. A better understanding of the effects of acute asphyxia has been obtained as a result of experimental work in animals. An initial period of tachypnoea and tachycardia is followed by a variable period of primary apnoea. If oxygen is administered at this stage it usually leads to the onset of regular respiration within a short period of time. If the asphyxia is allowed to continue, however, primary apnoea is followed by a series of gasping breaths which eventually stop as a severe mixed respiratory and metabolic acidosis develops, blood pressure decreases and cardiac rate slows. A period of terminal apnoea then ensues from which recovery can only be achieved by artificial ventilation with or without external cardiac massage (Fig. 6.1).

It is not always easy to decide in the newborn infant at birth whether apnoea is primary or terminal. The Apgar scoring system (Table 6.1) has been widely used as a method of assessing the infant's condition, a score of less than 4 being highly suggestive of terminal apnoea. *There is, however, a danger that resuscitation will be delayed in an attempt to assess the Apgar score correctly.* A simplified score based on heart rate at birth and the time taken for spontaneous respiratory movements to appear has been described by Chamberlain and Banks (1974) and may be just as useful. The possibility of fetal asphyxia developing at birth should be suspected in cases of fetal distress, prematurity, difficult forceps or breech delivery, twins (especially the second twin) and Rhesus incompatibility. Infants born by Caesarian section are also at risk. The situation may be complicated by the technique

Table 6.1 The Apgar score

	0	1	2
Colour	White	Blue	Pink
Heart rate	0	<100	>100
Activity in response to pharyngeal suction	Nil	Grimace	Cough
Respiration	Absent	Gasping or irregular	Regular or crying lustily
Muscle tone	Limp	Reduced, or normal with no active movements	Normal, with active movements

174

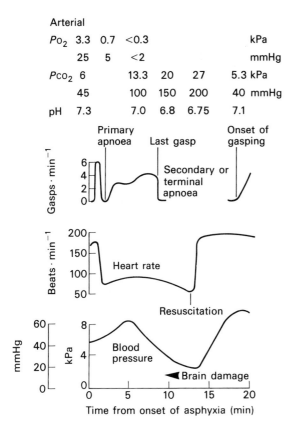

Fig. 6.1 Response to asphyxia and resuscitation by artificial ventilation in Rhesus monkeys. (Redrawn from Dawes, 1968)

of cord clamping. Early clamping is known to lead to hypovolaemia and this is associated with a higher incidence of respiratory distress syndrome (RDS). Birth asphyxia and late cord clamping are associated with a reduction in functional residual capacity, reduction in compliance, low arterial oxygen tension and high carbon dioxide tension. Since mortality from RDS is inversely proportional to gestational age, it is important to assess this as accurately as possible soon after birth. This assessment may influence decisions towards a relatively early intervention at birth.

Resuscitation technique

Immediately after delivery of the head, the infant's pharynx should be gently aspirated, though care must be taken not to touch the back of the pharynx as this may induce reflex apnoea. If central cyanosis is present, oxygen should be administered. The baby should be dried and quickly wrapped in a warm towel at birth and placed on a flat surface, preferably under a heating canopy because neonates lose heat rapidly during resuscitation. The temperature of the delivery room should be as high as can be tolerated by the staff, for the same reason. If the infant has not begun to breathe by 30 seconds after birth, a close-fitting face mask should be applied and the lungs gently inflated two or three times with oxygen. If there are no respiratory movements at the end of 1 minute or if the heart rate is less than 100 beats per minute at any time, endotracheal intubation should be performed and the lungs inflated to not more than 30 cmH$_2$O for approximately 1 second. This manoeuvre may instigate Head's reflex (p. 10), which is an encouraging sign that the baby is still in a state of primary apnoea and is often followed by the onset of regular spontaneous breathing. The first few breaths may be shallow and hard to detect but the tidal volume usually increases rapidly so that adequate gas exchange is established within 2 minutes. It is occasionally necessary to inflate the lungs with pressures slightly greater than 30 cmH$_2$O and pneumothorax is rare in this situation except in cases of pulmonary hypoplasia. If spontaneous breathing does not commence, intermittent positive pressure ventilation (IPPV) should be started at a rate of 15 times a minute. After the first inflation, care should be taken not to apply pressures higher than 30 cmH$_2$O to the airway. Inflating pressures of up to 60 cmH$_2$O can be achieved with high flow rates relatively easily even if a simple water manometer set at 30 cmH$_2$O is incorporated into the circuit.

If adequate expansion of the lungs is not achieved, the position of the endotracheal tube should be checked, as it may be in the oesophagus or in one of the bronchi. The stomach should be deflated by the passage of an intragastric tube. The most reliable sign of successful resuscitation is an increase in heart rate, which should usually exceed 100 beats per minute within 30 seconds of starting IPPV. If this does not occur, it suggests that the asphyxia is very severe and external cardiac massage should be commenced. The continued occurrence of occasional gasps after the onset of regular respiration should be viewed with suspicion, and if these continue for more than 30 minutes the possibility of intraventricular cerebral haemorrhage or metabolic acidosis should be considered. Gasps occurring without the onset of regular respiration suggest hypoplasia of the lungs. Gross hypoplasia is frequently associated with congenital diaphragmatic hernia and lesser degrees are seen in severe Rhesus incompatibility. In Potter's syndrome, pulmonary hypoplasia is associated with renal anomalies and peculiarities of the face, including large low-set ears and prominent facial creases.

Circulatory arrest

If the heart rate does not increase to more than 100 beats per minute within 1 minute of effective IPPV, external cardiac massage should be commenced. This can be carried out by slight pressure over the lower part of the sternum with two thumbs or two fingers (Fig. 6.2). If an effective circulation is not obtained within 3–4 minutes, it may be wise to give an intracardiac injection

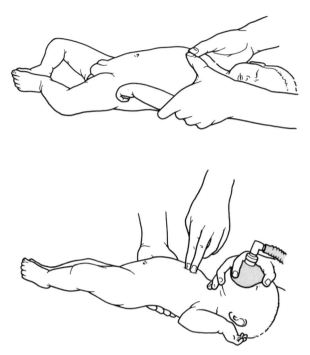

Fig. 6.2 Alternative positions of the hands for external cardiac massage in infants. (From Davenport and Valman, 1980)

of 2–4 mmol of sodium bicarbonate. Though the use of continuous infusions of glucose or bicarbonate has been suggested, there appears to be little evidence of their value.

Drug therapy

The empirical use of sodium bicarbonate has been mentioned above; if, after successful resuscitation, residual acidosis is suspected an arterial blood sample should be taken and base deficit corrected with bicarbonate according to the formula:

dose of bicarbonate = 0.3 × body weight × base deficit
(mmol)   (kg)

It is usual to commence with a half correction.

If the mother has received pethidine or morphine (Table 6.2) within 2 hours of delivery, a pharmacological antagonist can be given to the infant. Naloxone in an intramuscular dose of $0.005–0.01 \, mm \cdot kg^{-1}$ is suitable.

Since circulatory insufficiency immediately after birth is usually associated with severe bradycardia rather than ventricular fibrillation or asystole, myocardial stimulant drugs are seldom required.

Table 6.2 Drugs commonly given to mothers and their effects on fetus and neonate.

Drugs given to mother	Fetal and neonatal problems
Opiates	Respiratory depression. Premature infant achieves higher brain levels, and has retarded metabolism and diminished renal excretion
Pethidine	Respiratory depression. Breakdown products are also depressant and have a maximal effect between 2 and 3 hours
Tranquillizers	Additive to analgesic depression. Some sedatives cause hypothermia and prolonged hypotonia
Diazepam	Hypothermia and apnoea. Long half-life. May diminish normal fetal heart rate variation
Ultra-short-acting barbiturates	Least depression if less than 250 mg of thiopentone is used and 4–8 minutes elapse between induction and delivery
Nitrous oxide	Minimal depression that becomes worse with time of exposure. Neonatal pulmonary excretion could cause diffusion anoxia
Halothane	May abolish fetal heart rate distress patterns in low concentrations. Diabetic infants may become hypoglycaemic
Other vapours and cyclopropane	Minimal depression in carefully controlled analgesic levels
Neuromuscular blocking drugs	Gallamine easily transferred across the placenta. All require close control. Only pancuronium not yet detected in newborn
Local anaesthetics	Fetal bradycardia with overdose, paracervical block, accidental intravenous or fetal injection
Magnesium	Hypotonia and respiratory depression if maternal plasma level high
Alcohol	Acidosis, hypoglycaemia, CNS depression if grossly excessive amounts given

(From Davenport and Valman, 1980)

Prognosis

The Apgar score is of little prognostic value, and on the whole the outlook following recovery from a period of acute asphyxia is generally accepted to be good. Even delays of as long as 20 minutes in establishing spontaneous respiration in very low birth weight babies without cardiac arrest have been shown to have little influence on the eventual outcome. Low birth weight babies who require continuous IPPV for any length of time seldom survive the neonatal period, but for those who do the ultimate prognosis appears reasonable. There appears to be a high risk of permanent brain damage in any baby in whom regular spontaneous breathing is not established within 30 minutes of a period of circulatory arrest (Table 6.3). If, however, regular spontaneous breathing, as opposed to the intermittent gasping which may

Table 6.3 The prognosis for babies receiving cardiac massage for circulatory arrest within 15 minutes of birth

Time taken for regular spontaneous respiratory movements to develop after the circulation was restored	Outcome		
	Normal	Quadriplegia	Dead
≤ 30 min	26	0	2
> 30 min	1	9	12

(From Hey, 1977b)

occur in severe asphyxia, is established within 30 minutes the risk of cerebral damage is less.

The outlook following chronic intrapartum asphyxia is less certain. One group of babies have been identified who following intrapartum bradycardia and meconium-stained liquor develop problems of cardiorespiratory adaptation after delivery, with intractable persistence of the fetal circulation. The outlook for these babies can be improved by a combination of alkali therapy and artificial ventilation in an attempt to keep them mildly alkalotic, as this makes reversion to fetal circulation less likely. It seems reasonable to start the regimen early in this group. The presence of prolonged fetal distress or serious intrapartum haemorrhage appears to increase the risk of cerebral palsy, and as long as resuscitation is commenced within a few minutes of birth it seems that the likelihood of any eventual handicap is mainly determined by events occurring *in utero*.

Equipment

Equipment for cardiopulmonary resuscitation should be readily available at all times, and should be checked regularly to ensure that it is complete and reliable when required (Table 6.4).

Resuscitators

Although ventilation of the lungs can be performed with a T-piece, a certain amount of training is required, and it cannot be used in situations where there is no oxygen. A number of self-inflating resuscitators are commercially available which overcome these difficulties (Fig. 6.3). Any assessment of these resuscitators should include an evaluation of the ease with which they can be used, whether the state of the lungs can be determined by the 'feel' of an inflating bag, the maximum inspired oxygen fraction ($F_{I}o_2$) which can be achieved and the ease with which the resuscitator can be sterilized. Table 6.5 shows an evaluation of these factors for four commercially available resuscitators, together with the maximum pressure which could be achieved when inflating dummy lungs of compliance 1 and 5 ml·cmH$_2$O^{-1}. It also shows the length of time during which an inflating pressure can be sustained.

Table 6.4 Neonatal resuscitation equipment

Self-inflating resuscitator	Needles
Endotracheal tubes	Scalp vein needles
Tube connectors	Stethoscope
Laryngoscope	Scissors
Face mask	Umbilical catheters
Chest drain	Gastric tube
Suction catheters	Dextrostix
Syringes	

Drugs
Sodium bicarbonate—8.4 per cent
Adrenaline—1 : 10 000
Calcium chloride—10 mmol in 10 ml
Naloxone (Narcan)—0.01 mg·kg^{-1}
Water for injection
Saline
Dextrose—50 per cent (dilute to 12.5 per cent)
Heparin

There is still uncertainty regarding the pressures and frequencies at which the lungs should be ventilated during resuscitation. Unfortunately, what is adequate for most babies is insufficient for a few. Hey (1977b) suggests that an inflating pressure of 30 cmH$_2$O maintained for a little more than 1 second appears to be the best way of initiating aeration of the lungs, though he admits that slightly higher pressures may be required to expand them in some babies. Though there is evidence that excised lungs tend to rupture at autopsy when inflated above 30 cmH$_2$O, alveolar rupture and pneumo-thorax are seldom encountered in clinical practice during resuscitation, and the vigorous infant creates considerably higher transpleural pressure changes during crying. All the neonatal resuscitators assessed in Table 6.5 were capable of reaching the inflating pressures recommended by Hey when inflating a dummy lung of low compliance (1 ml·cmH$_2$O^{-1}) but some, particularly the Sherwood 'Samson' resuscitator, were unable to produce a sustained pressure. This resuscitator is designed specifically for newborns who have never breathed, and the operator is instructed to ventilate 'as hard and fast as possible'. This unusual technique is said to reduce the risk of pneumothorax, even when used by relatively untrained personnel, but it is not yet clear whether it produces adequate ventilation. It is not recommended for use outside the immediate newborn period.

The ability to produce a high Fio$_2$ is also important, and there is no evidence to suggest that a high Fio$_2$ for a short period immediately after birth produces retrolental fibroplasia. Resuscitators should also be supplied with a close-fitting face mask of appropriate size and terminate in a standard $^{15}/_{22}$ mm connector to allow attachment to a standard endotracheal tube adaptor.

Table 6.5 Assessment of the performance of four neonatal resuscitators when ventilating dummy lungs of compliance 5 ml·cmH$_2$O^{-1} and 1 ml·cmH$_2$O^{-1}

Make	Maximum inspiratory pressure (cmH$_2$O)		Sustained pressure (s)	Maximum FiO$_2$	Ease of use	'Feel' of the lungs	Sterilization
	Compliance = 5	Compliance = 1					
Ambu	100	142	1.5	0.8	++	++	+(120°C)
Penlon	76	130	0.5	0.9	++	+	+
Laerdal:							
With safety valve	40	52	0.5	1.0	++	+	+
Without safety valve	80	95	1.2	1.0	++	+	+
Samson	36	61	0	<0.6	+	0	Disposable

Table 6.6 The dimensions and resistance of Cole pattern endotracheal tubes without connectors

Tube	I.d. (mm) (tracheal end)	O.d. (mm) (tracheal end)	I.d. (mm) (connector end)	O.d. (mm) (connector end)	Resistance (cm $H_2O \cdot l^{-1} \cdot s^{-1}$) at flow (l·min⁻¹)		
					1	3	5
8 FG							
Warne (old design)	1.6	2.7	3.0	4.6	26	102	228
Warne (new design)	1.5	2.6	2.7	4.7	135	250	—
Rusch	1.4	2.6	4.2	6.6	78	450	—
10 FG							
Warne (old design)	2.1	3.4	3.0	5.0	34	44	62
Warne (new design)	1.9	3.3	3.3	5.3	54	84	120
Rusch	2.0	3.2	4.2	6.0	33	50	68
Portex 2.0 mm	2.2	3.5	3.7	5.4	35	38	52
12 FG							
Warne (old design)	2.7	4.0	4.0	5.9	10	16	19
Warne (new design)	2.5	4.0	4.0	6.4	21	32	47
Rusch	2.4	4.4	4.2	7.0	19	30	44
Portex 2.5 mm	2.7	4.0	3.7	5.4	13	20	23
14 FG							
Warne (old design)	3.0	4.7	4.4	6.5	8	11	15
Warne (new design)	2.8	4.3	4.5	6.6	12	20	22
Rusch	3.0	4.9	4.2	7.8	9	16	22
Portex 3.0 mm	3.0	4.7	5.1	7.0	7	12	16

(From Hatch, 1978)

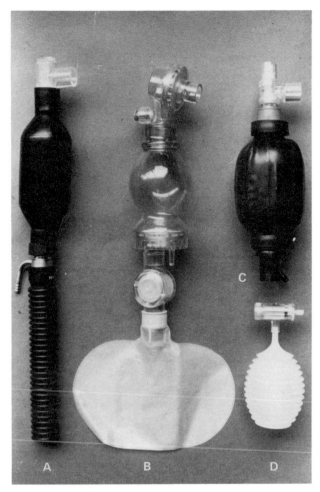

Fig. 6.3 Four neonatal resuscitators: A, Penlon; B, Vickers–Laerdal; C, Ambu; D, Samson.

Endotracheal tubes

Cole pattern endotracheal tubes are popular in neonatal resuscitation because of the ease with which they can be passed into the trachea by relatively untrained staff. The increase in diameter above the short tracheal portion of the tube makes endobronchial intubation unlikely, but the tube can be displaced into the oesophagus fairly easily. Because of the high incidence of laryngeal problems with oral tubes as opposed to nasal ones, many people prefer not to use them for prolonged airway management. It should also be remembered that the sudden change in diameter of these tubes causes turbulent flow even at low flow rates, with increased resistance to breathing (Figs. 6.4 and 6.5). For this reason the smallest Cole pattern tubes, which may have an internal diameter of little more than 1 mm, should not be used with spontaneous breathing for more than a few minutes (Table 6.6).

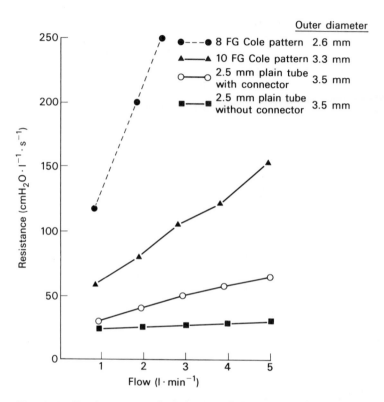

Fig. 6.4   Resistances of plain and Cole pattern endotracheal tubes.

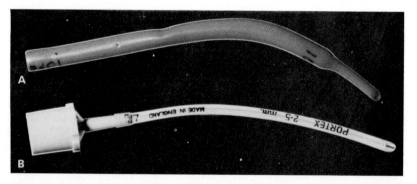

Fig. 6.5   The sudden change in diameter of a 10 FG Cole pattern tube (A) gives it a similar resistance to a 2.5 mm plain tube with connector (B).

Other resuscitation equipment

Resuscitation of the newborn is best performed on a firm surface of adequate height, with equipment readily available for oxygen administration, pharyngeal suction, endotracheal intubation and ventilation of the lungs. These conditions are provided by a resuscitation trolley such as the Resuscitaire (Fig. 6.6), which also incorporates an overhead heating canopy to minimize heat loss. A manometer to prevent excessive airway pressures being used during ventilation is essential.

Laryngoscopes and masks are discussed on p. 63.

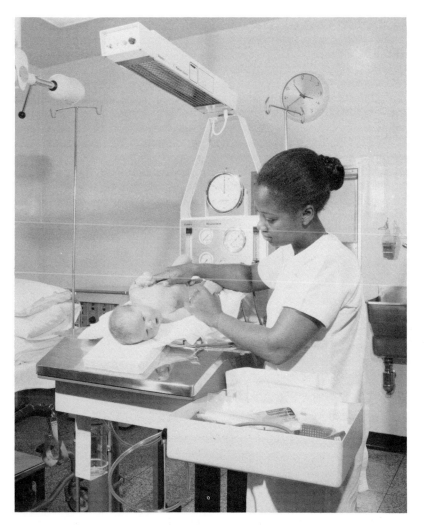

Fig. 6.6 The Vickers Resuscitaire.

References and further reading

Cave, P. and Fletcher, G. (1968). Resistance of nasotracheal tubes used in infants. *Anesthesiology* **29**, 588.

Chamberlain, G. and Banks, J. (1974). Assessment of the Apgar score. *Lancet* **ii**, 1225.

Davenport, H. T. and Valman, H. B. (1980). Resuscitation of the newborn. In: *General Anaesthesia*, 4th edn. Ed. by T. C. Gray, J. F. Nunn and J. E. Utting. Butterworths, London.

Godfrey, S. (1974). Growth and development of the respiratory system—functional development. In: *Scientific Foundations of Paediatrics*, Ed. by J. A. Davies and J. Dobbing. Heinemann Medical, London.

Hatch, D. J. (1978). Tracheal tubes and connectors used in neonates—dimensions and resistance to breathing. *British Journal of Anaesthesia* **50**, 959.

Hey, E. N. (1977a). The care of babies in incubators. In: *Recent Advances in Paediatrics, 4*. Ed. by D. Gairdner and D. Hull. Churchill Livingstone, Edinburgh and London.

Hey, E. N. (1977b). Resuscitation at birth. *British Journal of Anaesthesia* **49**, 25.

Hull, D. (1977). Lung expansion and ventilation during resuscitation of asphyxiated newborn infants. *Journal of Pediatrics* **75**, 47.

Samson, H. H. (1974). Resuscitation of the newborn—an improved neonatal resuscitator. *South African Medical Journal* **48**, 628.

Weiner, P. C., Hogg, M. I. J. and Rosen, M. (1977). Effects of naloxone on pethidine-induced neonatal depression. 1. Intravenous naloxone. 2. Intramuscular naloxone. *British Medical Journal* **2**, 229.

Appendix 1
Unusual medical conditions in the neonate with implications for the anaesthetist

Adrenogenital syndrome	Defect in hydrocortisone synthesis—need hydrocortisone Virilization of the female Electrolyte disturbances
Albright–Butler syndrome	Renal tubular acidosis Hypokalaemia
Analbuminaemia	Very low serum albumin Sensitive to drugs bound to albumin (e.g. curare)
Anderson's syndrome	Mid-facial hypoplasia Airway and intubation problems
Apert's syndrome	Hypertelorism Craniosynostosis May have congenital heart disease—antibiotics necessary Intubation difficulties
Arnold–Chiari syndrome	See p. 122
Arthrogryposis multiplex congenita	Congenital contractures Airway problems Difficult veins

Ataxia telangiectasia	Abnormal movements Telangiectasia of skin Defective immunity Sterile equipment and precautions Anaemia—correct preoperatively
Bartter's syndrome	Metabolic alkalosis and hypokalaemia Overproduction of prostaglandin E Poor response to noradrenaline Electrolyte abnormalities
Beckwith's syndrome (Beckwith–Wiedemann)	High birth weight Macroglossia, exomphalos—airway problems Persistent hypoglycaemia—careful monitoring
Bonnevie–Ullrich syndrome	Similar to Turner's syndrome Redundant skin of neck Congenital heart disease
Carpenter's syndrome	Characteristic facies Congenital heart disease—antibiotics necessary Mandibular hypoplasia—airway problems
Central core disease	Hypotonia Risk of malignant hyperpyrexia Poor respiratory function
Cerebrohepatorenal syndrome (Zellweger's syndrome)	Jaundice Renal failure Cardiac failure Hypotonia
Chediak–Higashi syndrome	Immunodeficiency; recurrent infections—need to use sterile techniques Thrombocytopenia
Chotzen's syndrome	Craniosynostosis Renal abnormalities with failure Difficult intubation
Cri-du-chat syndrome	Odd cry Microcephaly Hypertelorism Cleft palate Cardiac anomalies

Crouzon's disease	Craniosynostosis Hypertelorism Difficult intubation
Diastematomyelia	See p. 120
DiGeorge's syndrome	Absent thymus and parathyroids Immunodeficiency; recurrent infections Stridor Cardiac anomalies
Down's syndrome (trisomy 21)	Hypotonia Mental retardation Duodenal atresia Airway problems Cardiac anomalies; often atrioventricular defects
Edwards' syndrome (trisomy 18)	Most have heart disease Micrognathia Intubation difficulties
Ellis–van Creveld syndrome	Ectodermal defects; short extremities Congenital heart defects Poor lung function with chest abnormalities Abnormal maxilla Intubation difficulties
Epidermolysis bullosa	Blisters from minor trauma Avoid anaesthetic trauma to skin
Familial periodic paralysis	Weakness secondary to K^+ disturbance Care with muscle relaxants
Focal dermal hypoplasia (Goltz syndrome)	Papillomas of mucous membranes, especially of airway
Gangliosidosis, type I	Progressive neurological respiratory failure Early death
Glycogen storage disease: types I to VIII	*Features include:* Cardiac symptoms Hepatic symptoms; bleeding tendency Hypoglycaemia Skeletal muscles affected

Goldenhar syndrome	Mandibular hypoplasia—airway problems Congenital heart disease
Gorlin–Chaudry–Moss syndrome	Craniofacial dysostosis—difficult intubation Patent ductus arteriosus
Jervell–Lange–Nielsen syndrome (cardio-auditory)	Congenital deafness Cardiac conduction defects Sudden death
Jeune's syndrome (asphyxiating thoracic dystrophy)	Severe chest malformations—need mechanical ventilation Renal failure
Klippel–Feil syndrome	Fusion of cervical vertebrae—difficult intubation Cleft palate
Larsen's syndrome	Congenital joint dislocations Hydrocephalus Subglottic stenosis
18-Long arm deletion	Mental retardation Cleft palate Long hands Cardiac anomalies
Leopard syndrome	Hypertelorism—intubation difficulties Congenital heart disease Pulmonary stenosis Hypospadias Kyphoscoliosis; respiratory failure later Dark spots on the skin
Maple syrup urine disease	No metabolism of leucine, isoleucine and valine Hypoglycaemia Neurological damage Acidotic episodes
Meckel's syndrome	Microcephaly, micrognathia, left epiglottis Heart disease Renal dysplasia
Moebius' syndrome	Paralysis of VI and VII cranial nerves Micrognathia—difficult intubation Lung damage with recurrent aspiration

Mucopolysaccharidoses: types I to VII including Hurler and Hunter syndromes (gargoylism)	Intubation difficulty Cardiorespiratory failure
Myasthenia congenita	No relaxants
Myotonia dystrophica	Weakness and myotonia Cardiac arrhythmias Respiratory failure Suxamethonium causes myotonia
Noack's syndrome	Craniosynostosis—intubation difficulties Anomalies of digits
Noonan's syndrome	Micrognathia Failure to develop Cardiac anomalies Renal dysfunction
Oral–facial–digital syndrome	Cleft palate Mandibular and maxillary hypoplasia Hydrocephalus Polycystic kidneys
Patau's syndrome (trisomy 13)	Microcephaly and micrognathia Ventricular septal defect
Pierre Robin syndrome	Cleft palate Micrognathia and glossoptosis—intubation difficulties Congenital heart disease
Prader–Willi syndrome	Hypotonia Hypoglycaemia Absent reflexes Poor respiratory effort
Prune belly syndrome	Absent abdominal musculature Poor respiratory effort Renal anomalies
Radial aplasia–thrombocytopenia	Absent radius Thrombocytopenia Cardiac defects
Respiratory distress syndrome	See p. 45

Reye's syndrome	Liver failure Encephalopathy Respiratory failure
Riley–Day syndrome (familial dysautonomia)	Deficiency of dopamine-β-hydroxylase Autonomic instability Sensitivity to catecholamines Recurrent aspiration to lungs
Rubella syndrome	Mental retardation Deafness Cataract Interstitial pneumonia Osteolytic trabeculation in metaphyses Cardiac anomalies, especially ventricular septal defect
Smith–Lemli–Opitz syndrome	Microcephaly Skeletal anomalies with hypotonia and respiratory failure Increased susceptibility to infection
Treacher-Collins syndrome	Micrognathia and choanal atresia— intubation difficulties Heart disease Deafness
Turner's syndrome	XO females Web neck Micrognathia Congenital heart disease Renal anomaly
Vater syndrome	Vertebral anomalies Ventricular septal defect Anal atresia Tracheo-oesophageal fistula Radial dysplasia Renal anomalies
Werdnig–Hoffmann disease	Severe muscular atrophy Respiratory failure—resulting in early death
William's syndrome (infantile hypercalcaemia syndrome)	Mental retardation Coarse hair Aortic and pulmonary stenosis Characteristic facies

Wilson–Mikity syndrome	Prematurity Severe lung disease with fibrosis and cysts (aetiology unknown)
Wolff–Parkinson–White syndrome	ECG shows prolonged QRS Paroxysmal tachycardia and other arrhythmias Effects accentuated by neostigmine
Wolman's disease	Failure to thrive Xanthomatous infiltration of heart, liver, etc.

Appendix II
Guidelines for drug dosage in paediatric anaesthetic practice

All drugs are given on the basis of body weight (kg)

Premedication

Atropine   up to 2.5 kg   0.15 mg
             2.5–8 kg   0.2 mg   i.m. $\frac{3}{4}$ hour preoperatively

Injection pethidine compound (Inj. Peth. Co.)   0.07 **ml**·kg^{-1} i.m. $\frac{3}{4}$ hour preoperatively. (Used only before open heart surgery in the neonate.)

    1 ml contains: pethidine   25 mg
                     promethazine   6.25 mg
                     chlorpromazine 6.25 mg

For cardiac catheters, Peth. Co. up to 0.05 ml·kg^{-1} i.m. may be given $\frac{1}{2}$ hour before catheterization.

Anaesthetic agents

All are given intravenously unless stated otherwise.

Thiopentone	2 mg·kg^{-1}
Suxamethonium	1–2 mg·kg^{-1} 1 mg·kg^{-1} for intermittent use in neonates total dose up to 25 mg
Tubocurarine	0.2 mg·kg^{-1}; dilute to 0.25 mg·ml^{-1}
Pancuronium	0.06 mg·kg^{-1}; dilute to 0.2 mg·ml^{-1}

194

Atropine and neostigmine:
 atropine   0.025 mg·kg^{-1}
 neostigmine 0.05 mg·kg^{-1}

Ketamine:
 induction   2 mg·kg^{-1} i.v. (or 10 mg·kg^{-1} i.m.)
 maintenance 1 mg·kg^{-1} i.v.

Analgesics intraoperative—for cardiac anaesthesia only

Pethidine 1 mg·kg^{-1} (maximum dose)

Morphine 0.2 mg·kg^{-1}; up to 1 mg·kg^{-1} total dose for open heart surgery

Fentanyl Up to 10 μg·kg^{-1}

Antibiotics by i.m. or i.v. injection

Ampicillin	Up to 50 mg·kg^{-1}	6-hourly for severe infections
Cloxacillin	12.5 mg·kg^{-1}	6-hourly
Erythromycin	12.5 mg·kg^{-1}	8-hourly
Cephalothin	25 mg·kg^{-1}	6-hourly
Gentamicin	2 mg·kg^{-1}	8-hourly

Other drugs by i.v. injection unless stated otherwise

Chlorpromazine 1 mg increments up to 0.5 mg·kg^{-1}

Dexamethasone 0.25 mg·kg^{-1} i.v., then 0.1 mg·kg^{-1} 6-hourly i.m. for three doses
For cerebral oedema, up to 0.5 mg·kg^{-1}

Digoxin Total digitalizing dose: 0.05 mg·kg^{-1}
    one-third stat
    one-third 4–6 hours
    one-third 8–12 hours
Maintenance: one-tenth digitalizing dose b.i.d.
For premature babies, total dose: 0.03 mg·kg^{-1}

Droperidol 0.3 mg·kg^{-1}

Lasix 1 mg·kg^{-1}, repeatable

Mannitol Test dose: 0.5 g·kg^{-1}

Naloxone 10 μg·kg^{-1}

Phentolamine	Dilution to $1\,\text{mg}\cdot\text{ml}^{-1}$; increments of $0.5\,\text{mg}$ for desired result
Practolol	Dilution to $1\,\text{mg}\cdot\text{ml}^{-1}$; increments of $0.5\,\text{mg}$; maximum dose $0.5\,\text{mg}\cdot\text{kg}^{-1}$
Propranolol	Dilution to $0.1\,\text{mg}\cdot\text{ml}^{-1}$; increments of $0.05\,\text{mg}$; maximum dose $0.1\,\text{mg}\cdot\text{kg}^{-1}$
Sodium nitroprusside	$3\,\text{mg}\cdot\text{kg}^{-1}$ in $100\,\text{ml}$ of 5 per cent dextrose. Do not exceed $1\text{–}1.5\,\text{mg}\cdot\text{kg}^{-1}$ total dose in 24 hours
Tolazoline	$1\text{–}2\,\text{mg}\cdot\text{kg}^{-1}$ over 3 minutes; then infuse the same dose hourly
Vasoxine	Dilution to $0.5\,\text{mg}\cdot\text{ml}^{-1}$; careful increments of $0.25\,\text{mg}$ to achieve desired result

Postoperative agents NO ROUTINE ANALGESIA IS NECESSARY IN THE NEONATE

Codeine phosphate	$1\,\text{mg}\cdot\text{kg}^{-1}$	Do NOT give i.v. because it causes a severe fall in cardiac output
Pethidine	$1\,\text{mg}\cdot\text{kg}^{-1}$	i.m. or i.v. ⎫ TO BE USED
Papaveretum	$0.2\,\text{mg}\cdot\text{kg}^{-1}$	i.m. or i.v. ⎬ ONLY FOR PATIENTS ON
Morphine	$0.2\,\text{mg}\cdot\text{kg}^{-1}$	i.m. or i.v. ⎭ VENTILATORS
Phenobarbitone	$1\text{–}2\,\text{mg}\cdot\text{kg}^{-1}$	i.m. to control seizures (4-hourly if necessary)
Diazepam	$0.2\,\text{mg}\cdot\text{kg}^{-1}$	orally
Triclofos elixir BPC	$30\,\text{mg}\cdot\text{kg}^{-1}$	orally
Syrup of chloral	$30\,\text{mg}\cdot\text{kg}^{-1}$	orally
Promethazine	$0.5\text{–}1\,\text{mg}\cdot\text{kg}^{-1}$	orally

Inotropic agents DILUTIONS ONLY ARE GIVEN. The effect of administration must be monitored. The strength may be increased if fluid restriction is necessary. Start at a rate of 5–10 microdrops per minute ($= 5\text{–}10\,\text{ml}$ per hour)

Adrenaline	Up to $1\,\text{mg}$ in $100\,\text{ml}$ of 5 per cent dextrose ($1\,\text{ml}$ of $1:1000$ contains $1\,\text{mg}$)
Isoprenaline	Up to $1\,\text{mg}$ in $100\,\text{ml}$ of 5 per cent dextrose

Dopamine   6 mg·kg^{-1} in 100 ml of 5 per cent dextrose. Each
            microdrop per minute = 1 µg·kg^{-1} per minute
            At a dose not exceeding 10 µg·kg^{-1} per minute, there
            is no α-adrenergic action

Salbutamol 2.5–5 mg in 100 ml of 5 per cent dextrose; 3–5 microdrops
            as an initial dose

Appendix III
Normal physiological values in the neonate

	Neonate	Adult
Hb	18–25 g·dl^{-1}	15 g·dl^{-1}
PCV (haematocrit)	50–60 per cent	45 per cent
Blood volume	70–125 ml·kg^{-1}	70 ml·kg^{-1}
Extracellular fluid (percentage of body weight)	35 per cent	20 per cent
Water turnover per 24 hours (percentage of body weight)	15 per cent	9 per cent
Serum K$^+$	5–8 mmol·l^{-1}	3–5 mmol·l^{-1}
Na$^+$	136–143 mmol·l^{-1}	135–148 mmol·l^{-1}
Cl$^-$	96–107 mmol·l^{-1}	98–106 mmol·l^{-1}
HCO$_3^-$	20 mmol·l^{-1}	24 mmol·l^{-1}
Blood urea nitrogen	1.3–3.3 mmol·l^{-1}	6.6–8.6 mmol·l^{-1}
pH	7.35	7.40
$Pa\text{co}_2$	4.7 kPa (35 mmHg)	4.7–6.0 kPa (35–45 mmHg)
$Pa\text{o}_2$	9–10.7 kPa (65–80 mmHg)	10.7–12.7 kPa (80–95 mmHg)
Base excess	−5	0
Total bilirubin	100 μmol·l^{-1}	2–14 μmol·l^{-1}
Total Ca^{2+}	1.48–2.68 mmol·l^{-1}	2.13–2.6 mmol·l^{-1}
Mg^{2+}	0.7–1.1 mmol·l^{-1}	0.6–1.0 mmol·l^{-1}
Phosphate	1.15–2.8 mmol·l^{-1}	1.0–1.4 mmol·l^{-1}
Glucose	2.7–3.3 mmol·l^{-1}	2.4–5.3 mmol·l^{-1}
Total proteins	46–74 g·l^{-1}	60–80 g·l^{-1}
Albumin	36–54 g·l^{-1}	35–47 g·l^{-1}
Serum osmolarity	270–285 mOsm·l^{-1}	270–285 mOsm·l^{-1}
Urine osmolality	50–600 mOsm·l^{-1}	50–1400 mOsm·l^{-1}
Na$^+$	50 mmol·l^{-1}	30 mmol·l^{-1}
Specific gravity	1005–1020	1005–1035

Index

Index